PROFESSIONALS

PILATES
METHOD

Thanks to Fitness Professionals Ltd (www.fitpro.com) for supporting the Fitness Professionals series

Note

It is always the responsibility of the individual to assess his or her own fitness capability before participating in any training activity. Whilst every effort has been made to ensure the content of this book is as technically accurate as possible, neither the author nor the publishers can accept responsibility for any injury or loss sustained as a result of the use of this material.

First published 2008 by
A&C Black Publishers Ltd
38 Soho Square, London W1D 3HB
www.acblack.com

Copyright © 2008 Debbie Lawrence

ISBN 9780713684694

A CIP catalogue record for this book is available from the British Library.

Typeset in Berthold Baskerville Regular by Palimpsest Book Production Ltd, Grangemouth, Stirlingshire

Cover image © Jumpfoto/K. Vey
Inside photography © Grant Pritchard
Illustrations © Jeff Edwards, except p.40 and p.41 © Ron Dixon of Typetech and p.48 © Jean Ashley

Printed and bound in Spain by Graphycems

This book is produced using paper that is made from wood grown in managed, sustainable forests. It is natural, renewable and recyclable. The logging and manufacturing processes conform to the environmental regulations of the country of origin.

CONTENTS

PREFACE

'Whatever challenges life presents, may we face them with: the courage of the lion; the ferocity of the tiger; the beauty of the leopard; the grace of the panther; the playfulness of the kitten. Let us not forget that all the creatures and lifeforms that live on this planet are the source of our own nature. May we serve to preserve them all.'

Since 1983, I have worked in the fitness industry as a teacher of a range of exercise disciplines (exercise to music, gym, circuits, relaxation, aqua, stretch, core stability, and so on). I have worked as a lecturer, assessor and verifier for YMCA fitness Industry Training (1987–2002). I am also an External Verifier and technical writer for Central YMCA Qualifications and an evaluator for the Sector Skills Council – SkillsActive.

My introduction to Pilates happened by attending classes delivered by a Body Control instructor (2000). I then went on to attend the 'Pathway to Pilates' programme run by Fitness Professionals in conjunction with Body Control.

Since then I have trained with Modern Pilates (Northern Fitness).

I currently work as a freelance writer and continue to explore and experience different methods of exercising and moving the body. I deliver and assess a range of Teacher Education programmes (City and Guilds 7407 and PGCE/Cert. Ed) and hold a Masters degree in Post Compulsory Education and Training (1999). I am also a qualified counsellor and have been studying in the areas of mind, emotions, spirit, meditation and related disciplines – tai chi and yoga – since 1997.

The integrative model described in this book draws from my personal and professional studies. It aims to integrate my own experience and philosophy with the many exercise traditions and practices that ultimately inform my approach.

Debbie Lawrence

ACKNOWLEDGEMENTS

Writing never becomes easier, but it seems to get more interesting! I continue to find motivation from within that encourages me to know more and share more.

I am, as ever, thankful for the people I know who are prepared to read my work and contribute their time and feedback. A very special thank you to Louise Barnett (co-writer of GP Referral Schemes) for reading all the material and taking time to challenge ideas and ask questions to promote my thinking. Thanks also to Jean Ann Marnoch and Jeremy Patrickson (CYQ), Jill May (REPS), Cherry Baker (Modern Pilates), Christine North (Northern Fitness), Sandi Keane (Modern Pilates) and Lee Buck (SkillsActive, VTCT).

Thank you to the models Claire Miller, Jane Hull, Alex Carr, Sheena Gawler, Jo Southgate and Zoe Rose Wyatt. Thank you to Whiteoak Leisure Centre, Swanley, Kent, for hosting the photo shoot. Thank you to my partner, Joe, for being himself and for his support, encouragement, love and positive energy. Thanks also to the team at A&C Black.

ABOUT THIS BOOK

The National Occupational Standards (NOS) for Pilates in the UK were finally established in 2005. These have been approved by the Qualification and Curriculum Authority (QCA) and entitle instructors to enter on to the Register of Exercise Professionals (REPs) at Level 3 when qualified.

These nationally agreed standards were developed by collaboration between:

• The Sector Skills Council (SkillsActive)
• The Register of Exercise Professionals (REPs)
• A number of leading training providers for the Pilates Method
• Awarding bodies.

As a consequence of these developments, Central YMCA Qualifications (CYQ) developed their Level 3 Certificate in Teaching Mat Pilates. This certificate is offered within their existing qualification suite, which specialises in qualifications for exercise and fitness professionals. Training providers who wish to deliver this qualification have to meet the Centre Approval Criteria specified by CYQ. This includes providing evidence of:

• qualified teaching, assessing and verification staff
• effective management systems and procedures (equal opportunities, health and safety, accreditation of prior achievement and so on)
• scheme of work and lesson plans
• learning and teaching resources.

The assessment criteria and specifications (theory papers, case studies and observation checklists for practical teaching performance) are developed by CYQ and mapped by them to meet the National Occupational Standards and standardise assessment procedures. All centre approval applications are evaluated by a team of External Verifiers to quality assure the process.

The first training providers to be accredited to deliver this CYQ qualification include: Modern Pilates (Northern Fitness) and Pilates Training Solutions. *Note*: All qualifications certificated by awarding bodies are placed on the National Qualification Framework (NQF). Further information on CYQ awards and qualifications on the NQF can be obtained by contacting these bodies (website contacts are listed at the end of this book)

In addition, REPs has now accredited a number of reputable training providers (Body Control, Future Fit, for example) with entry to the register via the Industry Recognised Awards. Organisations who wish to deliver industry awards have to submit their learning materials, promotional materials, tutor resources, assessment criteria, and provide evidence of quality assured systems.

All submissions received by REPs are reviewed by an appointed panel of evaluators to quality assure the process. *Note*: Industry awards are not listed on the National Qualification Framework (NQF). (For further information on the industry awards, contact REPs. Their website is listed at the end of this book.)

Prior to these developments, the only qualification certificated by an awarding body was the OCR Level 2 Matwork Pilates, which entitled entry on to REPs at Level 2 – 'Exercise and Movement'.

The aim of this book is to explore and discuss some of the principles and concepts of the Pilates method, as reflected by the National Occupational Standards and the CYQ Level 3 Certificate in Mat Pilates syllabus. The aim is to enable the application of theoretical knowledge and concepts to the practical teaching environment. It is assumed that readers have knowledge of related anatomy and physiology equivalent to Level 2 of the NOS.

Part One introduces the Pilates method. It explains how the method has evolved and the key principles advocated by some of the different approaches and schools. It also applies the method to models of physical and total fitness.

Part Two reviews the structure and function of some of the skeletal and muscular structures that the method focuses on. These include: the spine, pelvic girdle, pelvic floor, shoulder girdle and their respective roles in stability. Section two also looks at posture and posture types, breathing, the mind, emotions and relaxation.

Part Three briefly introduces considerations for structuring a Pilates session and looks at other planning and teaching considerations. It introduces a model for analysing exercise safety and effectiveness. It also provides an introduction to the reported original 34 exercises and outlines which of the exercises covered in the book could help develop the flexibility and strength to perform these original and more advanced exercises.

INTRODUCTION TO THE PILATES METHOD

Part One provides an overview of the Pilates method. Chapter 1 offers a brief exploration of how the Pilates method has evolved and looks at the principles that underpin it. In chapters 2 and 3, the components of physical and total fitness are reviewed and discussed in relation to the Pilates method, respectively.

HISTORY, PHILOSOPHY AND
PRINCIPLES OF THE PILATES METHOD

1

Evolution of the method

The founder and 'name' behind the Pilates method was the German-born Joseph Pilates (1880-1967). He brought his training system to New York in 1926, where he ran his own studio between the 1920s and 1960s. Pilates originally called his system 'contrology'. He worked with and trained many people. It appears that most of his students had extensive backgrounds in dance and performing arts and many became his apprentices.

Pilates didn't try to formally establish (or patent) his training programme, with the exception of publication of his book *Return to Life through Contrology*, which outlines his philosophy and details 34 exercises that could be 'practised at home'. However, he has been described as being 'possessive of his method' and reluctant to 'entrust it to others' (Latey, 2001). Despite this, he trained many apprentices, some of whom went on to open their own schools. Thus, the name Pilates remains and the method has continued to be evolved, developed and cascaded down by apprentices of Pilates himself and by apprentices of his apprentices.

It appears that Pilates himself was constantly evolving his method in light of his experience, life situation, research and reflections on his teaching practice. One of Pilates' philosophies was to work with the individual and develop a programme to meet their needs. Consequently, he was constantly adapting his programmes

and exercises in response to the people in front of him, many of whom were dancers. Although some of the original exercises may be considered controversial by many exercise professionals, the Pilates method should work with the person in front of you, using the exercises and the philosophical principles as a foundation and guide. This emphasis on the individual is intended to develop and promote connection between mind, body and spirit.

The Pilates Method Alliance (2006:1) offer their position statement to reflect what is and what is not in their opinion Pilates. They propose that:

> *'Pilates exercise focuses on postural symmetry, breath control, abdominal strength, spine, pelvis and shoulder stabilisation, muscular flexibility, joint mobility and strengthening through the complete range of motion of all joints. Instead of isolating muscle groups, the whole body is trained, integrating the upper and lower extremities with the trunk.'*

In addition, they suggest that the method of instruction should continue to evolve as developments occur within the areas of scientific research and biomechanics. The PMA also assert that: 'Pilates is not performed in a pool, on a small or large ball or in combination with other forms of exercise and still called Pilates' (2006:3). They list the range of appropriate equipment that Pilates designed (Reformer, wunda chair, for instance).

2

However, the PMA acknowledge that: 'Today, it is acceptable to apply the principles of Pilates to all forms of movement, exercise and sports and daily life activities as Joseph intended.'

What follows is a potted history of the evolution of the Pilates method:

1880 – Joseph Pilates born in Düsseldorf, Germany.

As a child, suffers from rickets, asthma and rheumatic fever. Works hard to develop an exercise regime to improve own health. Undertakes a range of activities, including diving, gymnastics, skiing, boxing, self-defence, karate, yoga, and Zen meditation. As a teenager, poses for anatomy charts because his muscles are so clearly defined.

1912 – Pilates travels to England.

Works as a boxer, circus performer and self-defence instructor. During World War I, interned as an enemy alien. Uses this time to develop his training regime and share it with other camp members. Devises rehabilitation programmes for those injured during the war. Begins experimenting with bed springs attached to the end of beds to create resistance while bed-bound (the 'Cadillac', a bed with four posts, springs and hanging bars, and the 'Reformer', a sliding platform with strings attached, evolved from this early experimentation).

1919 – Returns to Germany after World War I.

Works with Rudolph Laban and is introduced to dance. (Laban's work provides the foundation knowledge for the Keep Fit Association (KFA) training programmes.) The German government asks him to train the German army. Pilates wants to train to heal not harm, so leaves for the USA.

1926 – Travels to America.

Meets and marries wife Clara. Founds New York studio and develops own method of exercise, which he names 'Contrology'. Writes his books, *Your Health* and *Return to Life through Contrology*. The latter lists 34 of his exercises for practice at home and describes his philosophy for his programme. Trains a number of apprentices who will go on to open their own schools and develop the method incorporating their own ideas (apprentices include Ron Fletcher, Carola Trier, Bob Fitzgerald, Bob Seed, Romana Krysanowski, and Eve Gentry).

1967 – Joseph Pilates dies.

Clara continues running the studio until her death in 1977.

From the late 1960s to the present day:

Alan Herdman visits New York in late 1960s to work with Carole Trier and Bob Fitzgerald. Herdman brings the method to London in early 1970s and develops his own school and apprenticeship system. Apprentices of Herdman's go on to develop their own schools (Dreas Reynecke, Gordon Thompson, Micheal King, Phil Latey, Penny Latey). Herdman writes *Pilates: Creating the Body You Want*, *The Gaia Busy Person's Guide to Pilates*, and *The Pilates Directory*. Herdman is a member of the working group that develops the National Occupational Standards (NOS) for Pilates in the UK.

In 1970, Romana Krysanowski becomes director of Pilates NY studio.

In 1973, Dreas Reyneke, a dancer with the Ballet Rambert, opens his own school in Notting Hill Gate, London. Reyneke goes on to write *Ultimate Pilates: Achieve the Perfect Body Shape*, along with other books and DVDs.

In 1977, Hana Jones is introduced to the Pilates method. Begins apprenticeship with Gordon Thomson in 1982. Member of the working group that develops the National Occupational Standards (NOS) for Pilates in the UK. Member of the teacher training committee for the Pilates Foundation (2006) with Dominique Jansen, Susanne Lahusen and Anne Marie H. Zulkahari.

In 1978, Penny Latey, a classical ballet dancer, discovers the Pilates method. Trains with Alan Herdman, Dreas Reyneke and Gordon Thompson. Moves to Australia in 1988 and develops own school. Later elected inaugural President of the Australian Pilates Method Association (1996). Works as co-ordinator and senior lecturer on the Graduate Certificate in Pilates Method at the University of Technology in Sydney. Goes on to write *Modern Pilates* (2001).

In 1980, Friedman and Eisen publish *The Pilates Method of Physical and Mental Conditioning*, which provides exercise descriptions based on the Pilates method and introduces the initial six fundamental principles of the method – concentration, control, centring, flowing movement, precision, breathing.

In 1982, Michael King, a dancer with the London School of Contemporary Dance, trains with Alan Herdman. Opens own Pilates school in connection with the Pineapple Dance Studios. Authors a number of books on the Pilates method. Later co-founds the Pilates Training Institute (1999) with Nuala Coombs and Malcolm Muirhead. A member of the working group that later develops the National Occupational Standards (NOS) for Pilates in the UK.

In 1983, Nuala Coombs begins as a client of the Pilates method. Goes on to co-found the Pilates Training Institute (1999) with Micheal King and Malcolm Muirhead. A member of the working group that develops the National Occupational Standards (NOS) for Pilates in the UK. Later co-authors *Pilates and Golf* (2005).

In 1984, Moira Merrithew, a principal dancer with the City Ballet of Toronto, studies the Pilates method in New York with Romana Krysanowski. Studies exercise science in response to a disc injury. Consults with physical therapists and sports medicine professionals to refine the method further. Develops own school – STOTT Pilates.

In 1991, Jane Parsons begins training using Pilates to recover from an injury. Trains in Toronto with Moira Merrithew. Invited by Moira to become first STOTT Pilates instructor in the UK. Later works as managing director of Active Pilates Ltd., running in conjunction with STOTT and YMCA fitness Industry Training from around 2002.

In 1992, Lynne Robinson is introduced to the Pilates method by Penny Latey in Sydney, Australia. Trains with Gordon Thompson. Later travels to UK and develops own school with Gordon Thompson – Body Control Pilates (1996). Writes numerous books, produces a number of DVDs and is a leading figure in creating the UK Pilates boom. A member of the working group that develops the National Occupational Standards (NOS) for Pilates in the UK.

In 1996, Pilates Foundation (UK) founded.

In 1999, Sandie Keane trains with Moira Merrithew (STOTT) in Toronto. Develops her own style, Chi Pilates, and writes her first book,

Pilates Incorporating Chi Principles. Later a Master trainer for chiball method and tutor trainer for Modern Pilates (UK) (2002). Publishes second book, *Pilates for Core Strength.* Works with Oriental Body Balance College (Lancashire) and Loumet Inc (Australia) to develop a rehabilitation programme.

In 1999, Pilates Institute co-founded by Michael King, Nuala Coombs and Malcolm Muirhead.

In 1999, Claire Worman trains with Body Control Pilates while studying osteopathy at Oxford University. Teams up with Belinda Buttery, a trainer with the Pilates Institute and trainer in Neuro-Linguistic Programming (NLP). Pilates Training Solutions (PTS) later developed by the pair (2003). PTS becomes one of the first UK centres accredited to offer the CYQ Level 3 Certificate in Mat Pilates (2005).

In 2000, OCR introduces Level 2 Matwork Pilates into their suite of qualifications. Entitles membership to REPs Level 2 – Exercise and Movement.

In 2001, national presenter Cherry Baker develops Modern Pilates (UK). Industry recognition includes: Fitness Instructor of the Year with Exercise England (1993/94) and Nominated for Commitment to Education – Exercise Professionals (2002). She created a series of workshops under the name of Abdominal Revolution (1997). Works with physiotherapists and authors Christopher Norris and Jenny Heron to develop Modern Pilates, based on the latest scientific research. Christopher Norris is one of the UK's most respected sports physiotherapists. With physiotherapist Sheila Done, develops Pilates for working with those suffering from Parkinson's disease and multiple sclerosis.

Develops standing Pilates (2002). Authors numerous books and presents Pilates DVDs. Modern Pilates becomes one of the first UK centres accredited to offer the CYQ Level 3 Certificate in Mat Pilates (2005).

In 2005, Sector Skills Council – SkillsActive – collaborates with industry leaders delivering the Pilates method and awarding bodies to develop the National Occupational Standards for Pilates. Central YMCA Qualifications develops Level 3 Qualification in Matwork Pilates.

Latey (2001:13) suggests that nowadays 'There are almost as many variations to the Pilates method as there are people who practise it'. She describes the development of three different styles:

• 1980s – American East Coast, American West Coast and British
• 1990s – Hard, soft, rehabilitative and Pilates-based exercises
• 2000s – Repertory approach and modern Pilates

The repertory approach follows the original exercises, being more dynamic and fast and with limited adaptations. Modern Pilates uses Joseph Pilates's original philosophy, but adapting the principles and, in addition, being influenced by other movement disciplines, developments in psychology and mental and emotional theories (Latey, 2001:14). It would be fair to say that this book follows more in the tradition of the Modern Pilates approach.

Note: A list of the texts and the website addresses of some of the different training schools that have informed the history presented in this book is given on pp. 194–196.

Principles of the traditional Pilates method

The traditional principles of the Pilates method as suggested by Friedman and Eisen, and listed and described by Latey (2001), include: concentration, control, centring, flowing movement, precision, breathing. A summary of the key features of each principle follows:

Concentration

This involves performing the exercises correctly and paying attention to all areas of the body, all the time.

Control

This means being in control of every movement that every part of the body makes – even little movements.

Centring

The central band of the body is the focus point and foundation for developing practice. Originally, this did not include the pelvic floor (Latey, 2001:11). Joseph Pilates' original method also recommended working with a flattened position of the spine rather than the 'neutral position' advocated by most modern approaches (PMA, 2006:2). STOTT (Merrithew, 2001) offers performing exercises with both legs raised, using a soft imprint initially and progressing to neutral. (The neutral and imprint positions are explained on p. 19).

Additionally, many of the original exercises involve flexion of the spine. However, changes in technology and lifestyle (work at computers, for example) have resulted in a greater proportion of people with a sedentary lifestyle, which involves a great amount of flexion at joints (hip, knees, spine and so on). Therefore, it is recommended by the PMA (2006:2) that a goal should be to be able to move the spine freely in all movement planes (rotation, lateral flexion/extension and extension, as well as flexion).

Flowing movement

This means moving smoothly and at a comfortable pace without jerking or stiffness to any movement.

Precision

This is defined as moving precisely and correctly.

Breathing

Pilates emphasised forced exhalation as the key to promoting fuller inhalation. His apprentice, Romana Kryzanowska, emphasised breathing in on the effort (Latey, 2001). This is contrary to what is practised by some modern approaches. Cherry Baker's Modern Pilates school suggests exhaling on the effort and that sometimes the eccentric phase may be the effort (Northern Fitness and Education, 2004). Body Control recommends that you 'breathe in to prepare, breathe out, engage centre and move and breathe in to recover' (Robinson, 2000).

In addition to this, the PMA (2006:2) promotes the use of costal breathing (sometimes referred to as lateral breathing), whereby the back and sides of the ribs move upwards and outwards during inhalation. They suggest that diaphragmatic breathing, which allows the abdominals to distend, should not be used for Pilates. Alternatively, Latey (2001:56) suggests that a diaphragmatic breathing technique can be used. Breathing techniques are explored further in chapter 8.

Principles of the Body Control method

Lynne Robinson, director of perhaps one of the most well-known schools – Body Control – further developed the original principles by removing control and precision and adding relaxation, alignment and co-ordination. So the eight principles proposed by the Body Control school comprise: relaxation, concentration, alignment, breathing, centring, co-ordination, flowing movements and stamina.

Relaxation

Relaxation is the starting point: 'Learning to recognise and release unwanted tension before you work out' (Robinson, 2000).

Concentration

This means being aware of how you are moving and focusing on each movement.

Alignment

This is correct postural alignment, which involves working primarily from a neutral position.

Breathing

This involves noticing how you breathe and trying to develop breathing that is wide and full and into the sides and back (Robinson, 2001).

Centring

This means stabilising the centre by engaging the pelvic floor and deep abdominals using the 'zip and hollow' technique (Robinson, 2000).

Co-ordination

Co-ordination builds on the five previous foundation principles and adds movement to aid learning and provide a base for further progression.

Flowing movements

This involves moving slowly with grace, control and lengthening away from the centre.

Stamina

Stamina means building endurance of the muscles by progressively challenging stability.

Modern Pilates (Australia)

Latey (2001) writes in support of schools removing the principles of precision and control by suggesting that attuning and connecting with the body is more sensible than bullying it through control. However, she also suggests that the addition of other principles, such as co-ordination, may require greater explanation (Latey, 2001).

In her approach, she offers nine principles: concentration, awareness, alignment, breathing, centring, precision, co-ordination, lengthening and persistence.

Concentration

Concentration is conscious control of movement by focusing inwards.

Awareness

This is defined as focusing on thinking, feeling and physical movement with attention but not domination.

Alignment

Alignment is developing a 'full understanding of the internal sense of equilibrium and gravity through movement' (Latey, 2001:19).

Breathing

Correct breathing will bring about other health benefits, with the breath being the 'interface between the outside and inside of the body' (Latey, 2001:20).

Centring

This means retraining the deep postural muscles to free up movement of the limbs (Latey, 2001:20).

Precision

Precision means practically applying the awareness of all body movements to achieve the fine-tuned control.

Co-ordination

Co-ordination is described as 'the unconscious grasp of complex sequentiality in fine muscle action to create flowing, global, emotionally connected whole body movements' (Latey, 2001:21).

Lengthening

This means elongating muscles and having flexibility to improve co-ordination, balance strength through the full range of motion and reduce stress on joints (Latey, 2001:21).

Persistence

Persistence is defined as perseverance, progressive practice and acceptance that there are no short cuts.

Base Line Essential Principles – Modern Pilates (UK) method

Cherry Baker's Modern Pilates school refers to the Base Line Essential Principles (BLEPS). These include bringing the individual's attention and focus to 'good posture and correct breathing in a variety of start positions' (Northern Fitness and Education, 2004:46). Consideration should be given to breathing, ribcage placement, abdominal hollowing, scapular stability, pelvis placement, neutral spine, and foot and leg placement.

Breathing

Breathing should promote oxygenation of the blood, improve circulation, promote relaxation and focus the mind. Lateral breathing into the sides and the back should be used, avoiding 'expanding the abdominal area and expanding the shoulders and top of the chest' (Northern Fitness and Education, 2004). Breathing out on the effort is encouraged, which runs contrary to the practice of Romana Kryzanowska, one of Pilates' original apprentices.

Ribcage placement

This involves softening the ribcage and maintaining connection between the abdominals and ribs.

Abdominal hollowing

This means engaging the core muscles that form a corset around the mid section by pulling upwards and inwards.

Scapular stability

Scapular stability means reducing the work on the upper trapezius by focusing on the movements of the upper body that enable the scapulae to glide over the ribcage.

Pelvis placement

This means selecting a neutral position for most exercises. The anterior superior iliac spine (ASIS) and posterior superior iliac spine (PSIS) should be level. Another way of gauging the position is to align the ASIS and pubis symphysis at the front, so they are level.

Neutral spine

This involves aligning the pelvis to create a natural curve of the spine. Norris (2001:10) describes neutral as being roughly halfway between hollow and flat, although he emphasises that this will vary slightly between individuals. As a guideline, he suggests being able to place the flat of the hand between the back and the floor (if you're lying down) or between the back and the wall (if you're standing).

Additionally, the STOTT method (Merrithew, 2001) suggests that consideration should be given for people with larger gluteal muscles. It is possible that for these individuals an excessive lordosis is created by trying to align the ASIS and pubic symphysis. Therefore, for some individuals, the main emphasis may need to be engage the abdominals, without trying to force the position and cause strain.

Imprint

Latey (2001:68) describes imprinting as it is explained by Eve Gentry: 'letting the bones of the spine relax into the mat as though leaving an imprint in the sand'.

Modern Pilates suggests the use of the soft imprint (slight posterior pelvic tilt to lengthen the lumbar spine) by lightly pressing (not forcing!) the vertebrae down towards the floor during exercises that elevate both feet from the floor. The STOTT method also recommends using an imprinted position initially (when both feet are elevated in an open kinetic chain) and progressing to neutral positions when sufficient strength has been developed (Merrithew, 2001).

Feet and leg positioning

As a general guideline, it's suggested that you keep your feet in line with your hips and knees, although variations for some exercises are offered. Many of the modern approaches pay greater attention to the alignment and positioning of the feet.

Thus far, it can be seen that there are many interpretations and developments of the original principles. To me, they all reflect the aim of connecting and co-ordinating work/ balance between mind, body and spirit and/or self that was a goal of Joseph Pilates' original method.

Integrating the principles – ABC

The aim here is to express and integrate the principles proposed thus far, without distorting their values, by using the ABC (DEF) approach – awareness, alignment, breathing, balance, centring, differentiation/development, endurance, flexibility. The following named principles may move away from those stated in the original Pilates method. However, it is hoped that they reflect the philosophy of passion, and the commitment to gather and apply knowledge to work with individuals and groups to develop the relationship between mind, body and spirit at a personal level, which may then extend outwards to relationships and connectedness to others and at a broader level – community and world (spiritual fitness).

Awareness

Awareness involves developing the concept of 'mindfulness' towards the body, mind and self during exercises.

It means being conscious and aware of, and attuned with, the way your body feels during static and dynamic posture. For example, you might notice the:

- Weight distribution between your feet when standing.
- Weight distribution of the body during other positions, for example supine lying, being on your hands and knees and so on.
- Changes in posture that occur during small mobility movements – for example, a shoulder raise, a heel raise, knee raise.
- The degree of contraction needed to maintain stability as the base of support reduces – for example, when you're standing, as you transfer weight from both legs to one leg; or when you're on all fours, as you transfer weight from both hands and knees to either one arm and both legs (raising one arm) and/or one arm and one leg (raising one arm and leg, as in a reciprocal reach).
- Changes in tension felt in the muscles.
- The position of the head in all start postures and during movement.
- The position of the shoulders in relation to the ears in all start postures and during movement.
- The position of the ribcage in relation to the pelvic girdle in all start positions and during movement.

- The engagement of the pelvic floor.
- The breathing, the pace of the breath, and the movement of the ribcage during breathing.
- The flow and pace of the movements.
- Any felt tightness and restrictions to movement (for instance, when stretching the hamstrings in a supine position, notice if the back wants to move out of neutral and push into the floor).
- Any felt weakness and instability to movement (for instance, when performing heel raises and knee extensions from the shoulder bridge, notice how transferring weight to one leg is experienced by both sides of the body).

In essence, awareness means developing a sensitivity towards the body and how it feels and responds and taking this forwards into everyday activities, for example:

- When standing in queues, taking the opportunity to align the posture.
- When sitting, taking time out to sit correctly.
- When walking, looking ahead rather than at the floor. I wonder how many kyphotic curvatures have been caused because of the tendency to look down at the floor rather than focusing ahead.
- Thinking about how the body is positioned when hoovering, lifting, carrying or performing other household tasks and daily duties.

Awareness from my perspective also means being aware of the activity processes within the mind during movement and stillness – and again transferring this awareness to other daily activities.

What are you thinking? Begin to notice the inner choir of voices:

The critical voice that reprimands your performance.

The nurturing voice that supports your performance.

The lazy voice that gets distracted and watches the clock.

The free child voice that enjoys the experience.

The competitive voice that seeks to compete with other class members and that thinks they should be progressing faster, rather than feeling the experience and comfortable limitations expressed by their own body.

The distracted and unfocused mind that is thinking of other things (the day at work, tomorrow's workload and a range of other thoughts they may be positive, negative or waste – all of which keep the mind active and not still).

The doom and gloom voice.

The positive 'you can do this voice' and the 'well done' voice.

In addition, awareness is connected to the self, which I will describe as our inner essence and power – the inner 'best friend'. The overactive mind and busy lifestyle distract focus away from this aspect. Stillness, relaxation and meditation enable reconnection. Many aspects of the Pilates method can assist with the development of this reconnection – for example, stillness and relaxation techniques, body and mind awareness and breathing.

Note: Developing awareness of body, mind and self is a lifelong process and needs continuous attention and patience.

Alignment – posture

Aligning the posture to provide an optimal start position and base for the performance of all other exercises and movements is essential. This includes alignment of the head and neck, shoulders and shoulder girdle, spine, ribcage, pelvic girdle, hips, knees, ankles, feet, elbows, wrists, and hands, in a full range of start positions, as shown below.

Standing posture

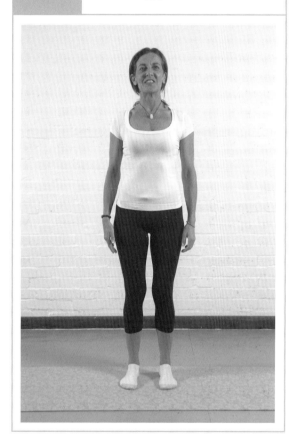

Fig. 1.1   **Standing posture**

- Stand with your feet underneath the pelvic bones, with your weight spread equally between both feet.
- Position your feet so that they are parallel to one another.
- Distribute the weight of your body across your feet (three-point distribution) – between the centre of your heel bone, underneath your big toe and underneath your little toe (where the toes meet the foot).
- Spread your toes.
- Align your second toe (the one next to your big toe) with your knee and pelvic bones.
- Find neutral pelvic position (pubic bone and hip bones in line vertically to ensure zero or minimal forward or backward tilt of pelvis).
- Ensure your knees are neither 'locked' nor bent, but soft.
- Lengthen your torso and neck.
- Engage the deeper abdominal muscles (so that the contraction can maintain the neutral pelvic position).
- Create a space between your pelvic bones and your ribs, without pushing your ribs forwards (maintain the connection of your ribs with your pelvis).
- Look directly forwards with your chin parallel to the floor.
- Keep your shoulders relaxed and down, with a space between your shoulders and your ears.
- Slide your shoulder blades down towards your buttocks.
- Open your chest.
- Place your hands by the side of your body with your middle finger level with the middle of your thigh. (The middle of your thigh is the line where the side seam of your trousers sits.)

Variation

Standing on *one* leg – alignment as above with your weight spread over one foot. Keep your pelvis level and avoid dropping your pelvis into your hip.

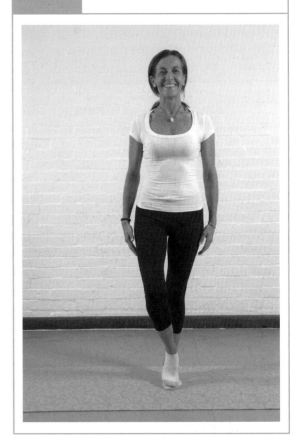

Fig. 1.2   Standing on one leg

Seated posture

Fig. 1.3	**Seated (chair) posture**

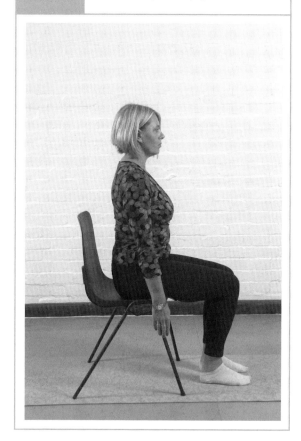

- Sit on a chair with your buttocks on the front third of the chair.
- Your feet should be at hip or pelvic bone width apart.
- Keep your feet parallel.
- Your knees should be in line with your feet and pelvic bones.
- Distribute your weight evenly across your feet (three-point distribution) between the centre of your heel bone, big toe and little toe (where your toes meet the foot).

- Spread your toes.
- Sit upright and lengthen your spine.
- Lift out of your sitting bones to find neutral pelvic position (pubic bone and hip bones in line to ensure zero or minimal forward or backward tilt of pelvis).
- Lengthen your torso and neck.
- Tighten your abdominals (so that the contraction can maintain a neutral pelvic position).
- Look directly forwards with your chin parallel to the floor.
- Keep your shoulders relaxed and down, with a space between your shoulders and ears.
- Slide your shoulder blades down towards your buttocks.
- Place your hands by the side of the chair, at the side of your body.
- Open your chest.

Note: There will be a slight, but normal change in the lordotic curve when in the seated position.

Fig. 1.4	**Seated (floor) posture**

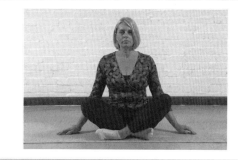

Variation

When sitting on the floor, it is recommended that blocks or wedges are used to facilitate correct alignment with different leg positions (extended, crossed, feet on floor). Sitting on the floor without the use of blocks demands great flexibility of the hamstrings and it can be impossible for a person with a flat back posture to achieve this position without the use of a block.

Kneeling posture

Fig. 1.5	**Kneeling posture**

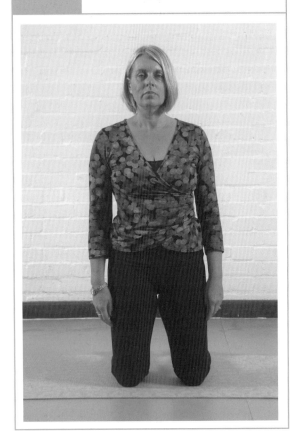

- Rest your knees on the floor with your lower leg flexed and buttocks lifted (not sitting on your heels).
- Ensure your pelvis is aligned over your knees.
- Ensure your knees are hips-width apart.
- Distribute the weight through your lower leg (not resting on your kneecap, or patella).
- Find neutral pelvic position (pubic bone and hip bones in line vertically to ensure zero or minimal forward or backward tilt of pelvis).
- Lengthen your torso and neck.
- Engage the deeper abdominal muscles (so that the contraction can maintain the neutral pelvic position).
- Create a space between your pelvic bones and your ribs, without pushing your ribs forwards (maintain the connection of your ribs with your pelvis).
- Look directly forwards with your chin parallel to the floor.
- Keep your shoulders relaxed and down, with a space between your shoulders and your ears.
- Slide your shoulder blades down towards your buttocks.
- Open your chest.
- Place your hands by the side of your body, with your middle finger level with the middle edge of your thigh.

Hands and knees posture

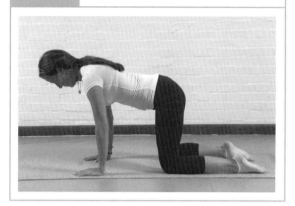

Fig. 1.6	Hands and knees posture

- Position your hands on the floor underneath your shoulders, and your knees on the floor underneath your hips.
- Spread your weight equally between these four points of support.
- Find neutral pelvic position (pubic bone and hip bones in line vertically to ensure zero or minimal forward or backward tilt of pelvis).

Note: Neutral position can be harder to find in this position as there are no contact points, such as the floor, for your spine to monitor and your hands are not free to check alignment. Alignment therefore needs to be developed by a felt sense. A strategy to assist finding neutral can be to move your pelvis to find first the flat back and then the hollow back, and then select a position between these two extremes.

- Lengthen your torso and neck.
- Engage the deeper abdominal muscles (so that the contraction can maintain the neutral pelvic position).

- Create a space between your pelvic bones and your ribs, without pushing your ribs forwards or downwards (maintain the connection of your ribs with your pelvis).
- Look directly between your hands.
- Lengthen your shoulders away from your ears.
- Slide your shoulder blades down towards your buttocks.
- Open your chest.

Supine crook lying posture

Fig. 1.7	**Supine crook lying posture**

- Lie down with your back on the floor, your knees bent (flexed) and your feet firmly on the floor.
- Ensure your feet and knees are in line with your hips.
- Distribute your weight evenly through your body and also across your feet (three-point distribution) between the centre of your heel bone, underneath your big toe and underneath your little toe (where your toes meet your foot).
- Spread your toes.
- Relax your hip flexor muscles.
- Find neutral pelvic position (pubic bone and hip bones in line vertically to ensure zero or minimal forward or backward tilt of pelvis).

Note: The STOTT method suggests that consideration should be given for people with larger gluteal muscles. It is possible that an excessive lordosis is created by trying to have the ASIS and pubic symphysis in line. Therefore, for some individuals the main emphasis may need to be engaging the abdominals, without trying to force the position and cause strain.

- Lengthen your torso and neck.
- Engage your deeper abdominal muscles (so that the contraction can maintain the neutral pelvic position).
- Create a space between your pelvic bones and your ribs, without pushing your ribs forwards (maintain the connection of your ribs with your pelvis).
- Look directly to the ceiling with your chin parallel.
- Keep your shoulders relaxed and down, with a space between your shoulders and your ears.
- Slide your shoulder blades down towards your buttocks.
- Open your chest.
- Place your hands by the side of your body.

Note: The use of a block or towel may help to facilitate correct alignment of the neck.

Side lying posture

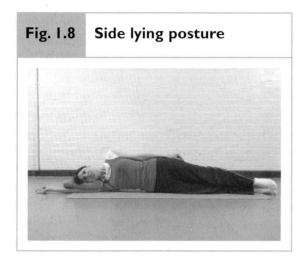

Fig. 1.8   Side lying posture

a space between your shoulders and your ears. (*Note*: If your arm is extended overhead just create as much space as is possible.)
- Slide your shoulder blades down towards your buttocks.
- Open your chest.
- Your top hand can rest on the floor or on a block in front of your body, or it can be placed on the top side of your body with the middle finger level with the middle of the thigh (the latter is less stable).

- Lie on one side of your body in a straight position. Your lower arm can either be extended overhead with your head resting on your arm and your palm facing upwards, or your arm can be extended in front of your body with a block underneath your head or ear.
- Your top or upper ankle bones, knees, hips and shoulders should be aligned with your lower limbs.
- Find neutral pelvic position (pubic bone and hip bones in line vertically to ensure zero or minimal forward or backward tilt of pelvis).
- Lengthen your torso and neck.
- Engage the deeper abdominal muscles (so that the contraction can maintain the neutral pelvic position).
- Create a space between your pelvic bones and ribs, without pushing your ribs forwards (maintain the connection of your ribs with your pelvis).
- Look directly forwards with your chin parallel.
- Keep your shoulders relaxed and down, with

Prone lying posture

| Fig. 1.9 | **Prone lying posture** |

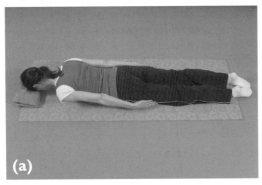

(a)

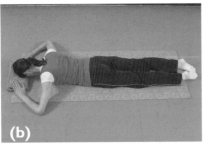

(b)

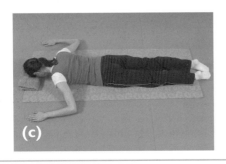

(c)

- Lie face down on the floor, with your forehead supported on a headrest to align your neck and enable your chin to maintain an alignment parallel to the wall at the feet end of the room.

- Your hands can rest in a lengthened position at the side of your body (Fig. 1.9a), or you can adopt a diamond shape with your hands at the side of your forehead and your elbows resting on the floor in line with your shoulders (Fig. 1.9b). You could also try placing your arms in a 'w' position, with your elbows bent out to the side of your body just below your armpits and your wrists aligned with your elbows (Fig. 1.9c).
- Keep your feet and knees in line with your hips.
- Find neutral pelvic position (in lean individuals the pubic bone and hip bones can be felt on the floor).
- Lengthen your torso and neck.
- Engage your deeper abdominal muscles by lifting your tummy button away from the floor towards your spine. This is so that the contraction can maintain the neutral pelvic position. It can help to visualise a small egg lying underneath your tummy button.
- Create a space between your pelvic bones and your ribs, without pushing your ribs forwards (maintain the connection of your ribs with your pelvis).
- Keep your shoulders relaxed and down, with a space between your shoulders and ears.
- Slide your shoulder blades down towards your buttocks.
- Open your chest.

Note: Depending on individual posture, it may be advisable to use a towel to enable some people to lie comfortably with correct alignment:

If people are inflexible around the ankles, a folded towel under the ankles may help.

A folded towel can also be used under the hips to lengthen the lumbar spine. This is useful if the position causes discomfort resulting from excessive lordosis.

A towel under the knees can help if an individual has knee problems (Keane, 2005:31).

Neutral pelvic and spine alignment: the base for performing exercises

The neutral spine position is one of the safest positions for the spine (Norris, 2001). It is the position where the natural curves are maintained to minimise stress on the spine and maximise balanced and equal muscular effort. Neutral position is considered to be halfway between a flat back and hollow back position (Norris, 2001). Neutral position is the key starting point for performing exercises safely.

Fig. 1.10   Pelvic tilt

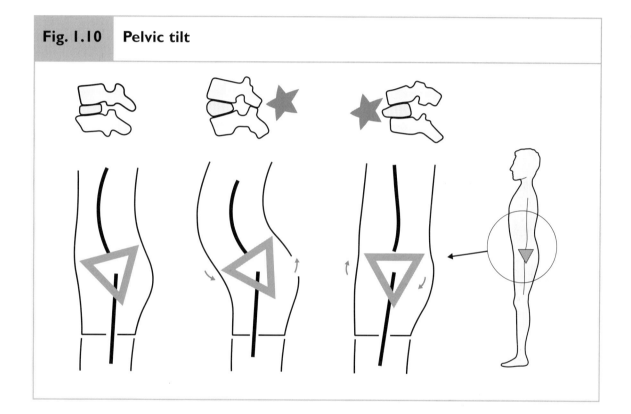

ACTIVITY: FINDING NEUTRAL SPINE POSITION

Start by either lying on the floor or standing against a wall. Tilt your pelvis to flatten your back; then tilt your pelvis to hollow your back. Repeat this a few times. Find a position midway between the two extremes – this is neutral.

Note: The flat of your hand should be able to rest between the wall or floor and the back. If the whole of your hand and wrist can pass under your back, your back is too hollow. If only your fingers can rest between the floor or wall and your back, your back is too flat.

Try these visualisations to assist teaching:

- Imagine a snooker triangle resting on your pelvis between the two hip bones, Anterior Superior Iliac Spine (ASIS) and the pubic bone. Visualise the triangle being full of marbles. As your back flattens, the marbles would roll towards your tummy button. As your back hollows, the marbles would roll between your legs. In neutral, the marbles would be still.
- Imagine a clock on your pelvis, with twelve o'clock at your tummy button, six o'clock at your pubic bone and three and nine o'clock at the sides on your pelvic bones (ASIS). An alternative is to use a compass (Robinson, 2000) with north at your tummy button, south at your pubic bone and east and west positioned on the right and left pelvic bones (ASIS) respectively.
- Place your hands on your pelvis, with heel of your hand positioned on your pelvic bones and your fingers pointing towards your pubic bones to feel the movement.

Note: It is advisable to develop awareness of neutral pelvic alignment in positions where the body is supported and the pelvis can be felt, for example, supine lying, where the floor provides a gauge for the movement, or, standing where the hands can be placed on the pelvis and/or a wall can be used. In prone lying, the pressure of the pelvis can be felt on the floor by leaner individuals.

The hands and knees and side lying postures are the most challenging in which to find neutral pelvis position. The individual needs sufficient kinaesthetic awareness to have a felt sense of the position.

Breathing

For relaxation exercises, abdominal breathing can be used. This is where the breath is taken into the abdominal region so that the abdominals rise on the inhalation and fall on the exhalation. This approach is not so practicable for moving exercises as the abdominal centre needs to be engaged (pulled in). For these exercises, a lateral or thoracic breathing technique is suggested. This is the same as that suggested by other schools whereby the breath is taken into the lower ribcage, expanding it to the side, rear and front (three dimensions). The upper ribcage is encouraged to relax.

Breathing will be explored further in chapter 8.

Balance

This is all about creating balance on a physical level between the physical structures of the body (involving muscle balance and skeletal alignment and breathing). It's also about creating balance on a deeper level – mentally and emotionally – and developing connections between the mind, emotions and body (awareness) to establish balance and gather understanding of how mental and emotional disturbances may manifest physically as health problems – stress, depression, high blood pressure, constipation, muscle tensions, and so on.

Core-centring

Core-centring means learning how to engage the core muscles that support the stability of the pelvic and shoulder girdle, and developing the strength of the stabilising muscles. A strong centre provides a foundation from which other exercises can be performed with precision and control.

Abdominal hollowing: engaging the abdominal core to stabilise the spine

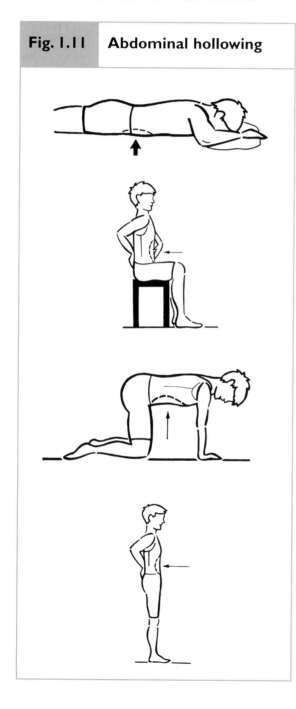

Fig. 1.11   **Abdominal hollowing**

Teaching points:

Keep your spine aligned and your pelvis in neutral position.

Breathe in to prepare.

Breathe out and engage your abdominal muscles by drawing your tummy button towards your spine – a 30 per cent contraction.

Keep your pelvis, spine and shoulders still.

Make sure your back doesn't flatten.

Keep your shoulders relaxed and your neck lengthened.

Note: Individuals should be encouraged to 'engage' the abdominals to a level appropriate to the specific exercise or activity. Initially people find it hard not to try too hard and may over-recruit and/or engage rectus abdominis, rather than transverses abdominis.

Progressions, adaptations and variations

The focus should be on raising awareness to engage the correct muscles (transverses) and also being aware of different strengths of contraction, which may need to vary for different exercises, depending on the leverage/resistance being used. Progression can be then achieved by performing in less stable positions (side lying and so on) and can progress to working with equipment.

Another method of teaching this is to have a piece of string tied around the tummy button and encourage pulling away from the string.

Alternatively, ask participants to hold the elasticated waist of their trousers slightly away from their tummy and allow the tummy to relax and fill the space. The abdominals can then be engaged (25-30 per cent) and the waist of the trousers released to provide a constant reminder (a felt pressure) for engaging the abdominals.

Visualisations to assist teaching:

- Imagine your pelvic bones (ASIS) drawing closer together like a concertina.
- Imagine your tummy button pulling backwards and upwards.
- Place your hands inside the pelvic bones (ASIS) and cough to feel the muscles that need to be contracting.
- Pull in maximally – 100 per cent initially, 50 per cent second time and 25-30 per cent third time – to develop awareness of the strength of contraction.
- Imagine zipping up a tight pair of trousers.
- Imagine a belt with ten notches. On the first contraction, tighten the belt to notch ten; on the second contraction, it to notch five; and on the third contraction, tighten to notch three.

Another teaching method I have used is to ask individuals to place their fingers on the fleshy part of the tummy, just inside the pelvic bones (ASIS), and 'cough' to feel the muscle engage. The aim of this is to raise awareness to transversus abdominis (TA) with the aim of reducing the work of rectus abdominis.

Differentiation/development

This principle involves being able to cater for different needs and abilities (offer alternatives, progressions and variations) within the same session, and embraces the concept of 'inclusion'. Layering information given to a group can enable inclusion of different levels and abilities within the session. Of course most instructors would prefer to offer courses for specific groups and this is perfectly acceptable. However, rarely even with groups labelled 'beginner' or 'advanced' are all participants of the same level and with the same needs.

In addition, most community learning programmes will require aspects of differentiation of learning to be included on schemes of work and lesson plans in order to accommodate different needs and meet the requirements of educational inspection bodies.

As a guideline only, the following levels are offered to differentiate between different abilities that may present:

Level 1

Apparently healthy persons who are beginners to exercise and to the Pilates method.

Persons with mobility conditions and/or other controlled medical conditions for whom some exercises may need to be modified further.

Level 2

Apparently healthy persons and persons with controlled and low-risk medical conditions who have some experience of exercise and are familiar and competent with the basic ABC principles in the full range of start positions.

Level 3

Apparently healthy persons who are fully familiar with ABC principles and competent to perform these in a range of start positions, with experience of all basic exercises and a developed level of endurance.

Level 4

Apparently healthy persons with a high level of strength and flexibility. Individuals who are fully competent with a range of exercises in the progressed forms. Individuals who require athletic challenge. *Note*: It is these individuals who may wish to progress to some of the original exercises. The practice of the more advanced, traditional exercises is not explored in great depth in this book. They are introduced briefly in chapter 12 with reference to the modified versions that are listed in this book. Level 4 individuals wishing to explore the traditional exercises should be advised to attend a specialist studio.

Note: The levels listed here are used later to suggest the appropriateness of certain exercises. Instructors should always use their knowledge and skills to adapt the exercises listed to match the ability of the individual. This can be done by using the intensity principle of training – repetitions, rate, resistance, range of motion and rest. These are discussed in relation to specific components of fitness in chapter 2.

Endurance

Once the ABC principles are established, basic endurance exercises can be introduced. A guideline is to start with more isolated and simple movements that match the individual's stability and build repetitions and endurance here before progressing to more complex and combined movements. Further progression of the exercise positions can be achieved by applying the principles of training for other methods of exercise:

Range of motion (smaller to larger); Resistance (shorter to longer levers and stable to less stable positions); Rate (working at a comfortable speed and developing pace – not too fast); Rest (longer rests will occur naturally in the beginner stages to teach the initial ABC principles. This can reduce over time as fewer explanations are needed); Repetitions (developing endurance again when one of the above progressions has been added).

Flexibility

This involves using stretching exercises within the programme to develop and build the flexibility and mobility of muscles around the pelvic and shoulder girdle. If these muscles aren't sufficiently mobile, movement can be restricted and other muscles can be over-recruited, reducing stability in these areas.

The original exercises were targeted to develop flexibility and many can do exactly that (these exercises are introduced in chapter 12). However, individuals need a good range of motion to get into some of the original positions (remember Pilates worked with a lot of dancers). Therefore, the more modest approach of including some simple stretches is suggested. Stretches for the key muscles affecting the range of motion of particular areas (spine, pelvic girdle, shoulder girdle) are illustrated and explained in specific chapters in part two of this book. Stretches relating to the flexibility aims of the original exercises are suggested in chapter 12.

PHYSICAL FITNESS AND THE PILATES METHOD

Physical fitness is one of the seven components that provide a model for total fitness and health. It can be achieved by performing specific types of exercise and activity in a structured format, at a recommended frequency (number of sessions/ activities per week), intensity (difficulty of the session/activity) and duration/time (the length of the session/activity). There are five components of physical fitness:

- Cardiovascular fitness
- Flexibility
- Muscular strength ⎫ muscular
- Muscular endurance ⎬ fitness
- Motor fitness.

Cardiovascular fitness

Cardiovascular or aerobic fitness is the ability of the heart, lungs and circulatory system to take in, transport and utilise oxygen and remove waste products efficiently.

Benefits of cardiovascular training

Regular cardiovascular exercise and activity is essential for maintaining health and quality of life. Cardiovascular exercise (walking, running, swimming, for example) strengthens the heart, enabling a greater volume of blood to be pumped in each beat (stroke volume). The capillary network in the muscles and lungs increases and there is also an increase in the size and number of the cells in which aerobic energy is produced (mitochondria) in the muscles. This combination of effects enables the increased transportation and utilisation of oxygen and removal of waste products (as lactic acid).

Low cardiovascular fitness and activity levels are associated with the increased risk of chronic diseases that are linked with coronary heart disease (diabetes, high blood pressure, and so on). Increased physical activity and exercise targeted to improve cardiovascular fitness can assist with the prevention of these diseases and promote longevity and greater quality of life.

Recommended training guidelines for developing and maintaining cardiovascular fitness are listed in table 2.1.

Table 2.1	Recommended training guidelines for cardiovascular fitness
Frequency	3 to 5 times a week. 3 times a week is sufficient for people exercising at higher intensities. More than 3 times a week is recommended for people exercising at low levels of intensity. Rest days should be alternated between vigorous training days. Vary the activities and cross train to alter the impact and so reduce the risk of injury to the muscles and joints.
Intensity	Between 55/65% to 90% of MHR (maximal heart rate). A range of 70-85% MHR is sufficient for most individuals when performed at an appropriate frequency and duration. Lower levels of intensity are appropriate for less active people; however duration may need to be increased.
Time/ duration	Between 20 to 60 minutes of continuous or intermittent activity, e.g. accumulating 10-minute bouts throughout the day. Minimum duration to improve cardiovascular fitness in apparently healthy adults is 20–30 minutes. All durations exclude necessary time for warm-up and cool down. Less fit groups will need to progress gradually to increased durations.
Type/mode/ specificity	Rhythmical, continuous activities that use large muscle groups. For example: walking, swimming, running, cycling, dancing, exercise to music, exercise in water, step classes, line dancing and the use of cardiovascular machines (rowing, stepper, cross trainer, treadmill, bike and so on).

Adapted from ACSM 2005 and Lawrence and Barnett, *GP Referral Schemes* (2006)

Inactive and less fit persons can start developing their cardiovascular fitness by working towards the Department of Health (2005) recommendations for physical activity to maintain general health. These targets are outlined in table 2.2.

Table 2.2	Physical activity targets for health
Frequency	Work towards building activity into daily routine on **5 days of the week (minimum)**.
Intensity	Work at a moderate level where you **feel mildly breathless, warm but comfortable**.
Time	Work towards performing the chosen activities for a total of **30 minutes**. This can be broken down and accumulated, for example: **3 x 10 minute** slots of activity each day; **2 x 15 minute** slots of activity each day.
Type	Any activity that fits well into your daily lifestyle! For example: • Walking to the station • Walking the kids to school • Vigorous heavy housework • Cleaning the car • Walking up and down stairs more frequently • Dancing to a piece of music at home • Active hobbies • Structured exercise and sporting activities • A combination of activity, exercise and sport. This recommendation can be tailored specifically to the lifestyle, preference and needs of the individual and is particularly relevant for people who find it easier and more acceptable to increase physical activity by incorporating it into their everyday life.

From Lawrence and Barnett, *GP Referral Schemes* (2006)

Cardiovascular training and the Pilates method

Pilates-based exercises in isolation provide little benefit for improving the cardiovascular component of fitness. Pilates doesn't include the continuous, rhythmic, sustained activities using large muscle groups that are needed to elevate the heart rate into the training zone to meet either the ACSM or Department of Health intensity targets listed in the tables above.

However, Pilates does focus on breathing and moving correctly and efficiently. Learning to breathe more fully and move more efficiently are transferable skills that can be practised during other activities. This may indeed be useful for enhancing performance during these activities, which in turn could elicit greater benefits in other areas.

It is therefore recommended that Pilates participants are encouraged to engage in other forms of exercise and activity that will bring about more directly the essential benefits of cardiovascular exercise (a stronger heart, for example). Any exercise or activity that uses the larger muscle groups rhythmically and continuously for an appropriate frequency, intensity and duration, such as those described in tables 2.1 and 2.2, are suitable for most individuals.

In addition, concepts that are focused on by the Pilates method should ideally be taken by individuals (and teachers) into the other forms of exercise they perform or teach, and indeed into their daily activities. For example, moving with correct posture, alignment and stability, breathing correctly and focusing on the movement being performed are essential for all forms of exercise (for example, step, weight training, exercise in water) and also for lifestyle activities (such as sitting at a desk, walking, gardening, lifting, and hoovering). Integrating the concepts learned into daily activities extends the benefits from attending a single Pilates exercise session.

Flexibility

Flexibility or suppleness is the ability of the joints and muscles to move through their full potential range of movement. A muscle is considered to be stretching (lengthening) when the two points of muscle attachment (the origin and insertion, or two ends of the muscle) move further apart and the muscle relaxes in that extended position.

Benefits of flexibility

Being able to move joints and muscles through their full potential range of motion is essential for performing a number of daily activities and tasks. Flexibility of the shoulder joint is needed to reach upwards to change a light bulb and pick objects from a high shelf and to reach forwards to button shirts and cardigans. Flexibility of the hip joint is needed to raise the knees to climb stairs and to take long strides when walking. Mobility of the spine and neck enables us to twist and turn and look behind us and to the right and left.

Flexible muscles and joints are essential for maintaining correct posture and joint alignment. Flexible chest and shoulder muscles (pectorals and anterior deltoids), and stronger muscles in the upper back (trapezius and rhomboids), help to prevent kyphosis (rounding/hunching of the upper back). Flexible back muscles (erector spinae), hamstrings and hip flexors, and strong abdominals, help to prevent the postural condition – lordosis (hollowing of the lower spine). Improved posture can potentially enhance physical appearance, reduce the incidence of lower back pain and assist with the management of joint mobility conditions such as osteoarthritis and rheumatoid arthritis.

Being sufficiently flexible contributes to an enhanced quality of life and reduces the risk of injury, especially for older people. It can also assist with relaxation and managing stress and tension in the body. The recommended training guidelines for improving and maintaining flexibility are listed in table 2.3.

Table 2.3	Recommended guidelines for training flexibility
Frequency	A minimum of 2 to 3 times per week. Ideally 5 to 7 days a week. The body must be *warm* prior to stretching to prevent muscle tearing and to enhance the range of motion.
Intensity	Stretch positions should be taken to a point of mild tension (stretch reflex), not discomfort, and held for an extended period of time once the muscle has relaxed (desensitisation). 2 to 4 repetitions can be performed for each stretch.
Time/ duration	Hold static for 15 to 30 seconds.
Type/mode/ specificity	Static stretches are recommended for the general population.

Adapted from ACSM 2005 and Lawrence and Barnett, *GP Referral Schemes* (2006)

Flexibility training and the Pilates method

Exercises that develop mobility and flexibility play an integral role within a Pilates programme. Joint mobility exercises are essential for obtaining a full range of movement at specific joint areas. Flexibility exercises that are targeted to lengthen shortened or tightened muscles are essential for making improvements to posture.

Note: Some tightened muscles may not necessarily be shortened or need lengthening. It may be that instead, *other* muscles need strengthening or postural changes are necessary to enable the 'tightened – overactive' muscles to 'let go'. For example, a lordotic posture may lead to tightened hamstring muscles, which are not necessarily shortened. In this case, it may be more appropriate to practise finding a neutral spine and to strengthen the abdominals.

Many of Pilates' original exercises were devised to improve flexibility. However, because Pilates worked with dancers, a number of the exercises demand great levels of flexibility to perform. Many of these are not be suitable for people who lack flexibility. The inclusion of more basic mobility and flexibility exercises is therefore recommended and encouraged for less flexible individuals.

When working with clients on a one-to-one basis, you can focus on stretching the muscles that are shortened. However, within a group there may be a variety of people with very different postural deviations. In this instance, a range of stretches may be necessary (whole body approach). See the section on posture in chapter 7, which explores muscles that may be inflexible in certain posture types. Proprioceptive neuromuscular facilitation (PNF) can be used by experienced trainers when working on a one-to-one basis with clients.

To maintain flexibility, the muscles worked should be stretched when they have finished working. This can occur at the end of the session, or in between exercises if the muscle is not going to be used again in the session. Stretching should always be performed when the muscles are warm to avoid injury. The muscle should be slowly lengthened to the end of the range of movement, to a point of tightness but not discomfort, so that the muscle can relax. This position is then held for up to 15 to 20 seconds (as long as is comfortable).

Static, developmental stretching should be included to improve flexibility. This can be achieved by taking the muscle to the point of mild tension, allowing it to relax and then moving further into the stretch (increasing the range of motion). The muscle tension (stretch reflex) will increase again and will therefore need to relax again. The extended position can be held for between 15 and 30 seconds or longer if comfortable and provided the muscle is very warm. These stretches can be repeated two to four times.

Progressing flexibility exercises

Inactive people and people with specific joint, muscular and postural problems may lack flexibility and will therefore need more supportive and comfortable positions in which to stretch. They may also have less body awareness and their exercise technique may demand more careful attention from the teacher (observation, correction, teaching) to enable safe and effective performance.

Range of motion, balance and isolation

The range of motion performed in mobility and stretching exercises can be progressive to meet the needs of the individual. Less flexible participants will generally need to work through a smaller range of motion, use more supported positions to assist balance and isolate the muscles being stretched (one muscle at a time as opposed to using compound stretches or more than one muscle at a time).

Floor-based stretches provide support to the weight of the body and can offer a more relaxed way of stretching. Using straps to support levers (quadriceps and hamstring stretch) and trainer-assisted stretches (PNF) can assist the range of motion and stretch achieved (see illustration 2.1). The key thing is to find the most comfortable and supportive position for the individual. *Note*: Use blocks or wedges for seated floor positions to facilitate effective seated posture in people with limited flexibility, for example shortened hamstrings.

Muscular fitness (strength and endurance)

Muscular fitness is a combination of, and a balance between, muscular strength and muscular endurance. It represents the functional fitness needed to maintain correct posture and perform daily activities. Muscular strength is the ability of our muscles to exert a near maximal force to lift a resistance. Muscular endurance requires a less maximal force to be exerted, but needs the muscle contraction to be maintained for a longer duration.

Benefits of muscular fitness training (strength and endurance)

Muscles need to be strong enough and have sufficient endurance to carry out daily tasks, which require us to lift, carry, pull, or push a resistance. This includes the resistance of moving the body when walking, climbing stairs, sitting down into, and rising up from, a chair, carrying shopping, gardening, moving furniture, and so on.

Strong muscles help to maintain posture and the correct alignment of the skeleton.

Weakened muscles may cause an uneven pull to be placed on our skeleton. The muscles work in pairs (as one contracts and works, the opposite muscle relaxes). Therefore, any imbalance in workload (if one of the pair is contracted or worked too frequently and becomes too strong or overactive and the other is not worked sufficiently or is allowed to become weaker or lengthened) will cause the joints (including the spine, pelvic and shoulder girdle) to be pulled out of the correct alignment. This may potentially cause injury, and/or create postural deviations such as rounded shoulders or excessive curvatures of the spine.

Some more common postural deviations are discussed and illustrated in chapter 7. To introduce these briefly, an imbalance of strength between the abdominal and opposing muscles of the back (the erector spinae) can cause an exaggerated curve or hollowing of the lumbar vertebrae (lordosis). Imbalance of strength between the muscles of the chest (the pectorals) and the muscles between the shoulder blades (the rhomboids and trapezius) can cause rounded shoulders and a humping of the thoracic spine (kyphosis).

All muscles should therefore be kept sufficiently strong to maintain a correct posture. Exercise recommendations when working with clients with specific postural conditions are discussed in chapter 7.

Training for muscular fitness will improve the tone of our muscles and provide a firmer and more shapely appearance. This can contribute to a positive self-image and can enhance psychological well-being and self-confidence.

Muscular fitness also improves the strength and health of our bones and joints. The muscles have to contract and pull against the bones to create movement. In response, our tendons, which attach the muscles to the bone across the joint, and our ligaments, which attach bone to bone across the joint, will become stronger. Therefore, in the long term our joints will become stronger, more stable, and at less risk from injury. In addition, increased calcium can be deposited and stored by the bones. This can prevent them from becoming brittle and reduce the risk of osteoporosis. The recommended training guidelines for developing and improving muscular fitness are listed in table 2.4.

Table 2.4	Recommended guidelines for training muscular fitness
Frequency	2 to 3 times per week (same muscle groups). Alternate rest days and training days (don't train the same muscle group on consecutive days).
Intensity	To the point of near fatigue, while maintaining good technique. For people with health conditions, finish the exercise when the lifting (concentric, or muscle shortening) phase becomes difficult, while maintaining good technique.
Time/ duration	One set of 3–20 repetitions. Choose a range of repetitions, e.g. 3–5, 10–12, 12–15. One set of 8–12 (high intensity) will elicit strength and endurance benefits for healthy populations. One set of 10–15 (moderate intensity) is recommended for older adults. Training time will vary depending on the level of fitness, number of exercises, muscle groups and fitness goals.
Type/mode/ specificity	8–10 exercises targeting the main muscle groups. Choose activities that are comfortable throughout the range of movement: • Body weight exercises • Free weights (dumbbells and barbells) • Exercise bands

Adapted from ACSM 2005 and Lawrence and Barnett, *GP Referral Schemes* (2006)

Muscular fitness training applied to the Pilates method

Creating and regaining muscle balance is an integral part of Pilates method training. In particular, regaining the strength of the core stabiliser muscles minimises overreliance on the movement – or mobiliser – muscles to work in a stabilising role. Mobiliser muscles tend towards increased tone and as a result can be used preferentially over the core stabilisers. However, they tire quickly and are less efficient at maintaining stability. Some muscles may act as stabilisers in one situation and as mobilisers in another situation. For example, quadratus lumborum (see chapter 4) acts as a stabiliser of the pelvic girdle and lumbar spine and also has a mobiliser role when the spine is laterally flexing.

Table 2.5	Stability and mobiliser muscles
Stabiliser muscles Examples: 　Transversus abdominis 　Multifidus 　Quadratus lumborum 　Gluteus medius 　Vastus medialis 　Serratus anterior 　Lower trapezius	**Mobiliser muscles** Examples: 　Rectus abdominis 　Erector spinae 　External obliques 　Iliopsoas 　Rectus femoris 　Hamstrings 　Upper trapezius
Tend to be deep (closer to the core of the body)	Tend to be more superficial (closer to the surface of the body)
Cross over and stabilise single joints	Cross over and move two joints
Most active in closed chain movement. Closed chain is where the end of the limb is fixed, not allowing movement. For example chin up (hands are fixed), squats (feet are fixed), press-ups (hands are fixed).	Most active in open chain movement. Open chain is where the end of the limb is not fixed, for example lat pull down, leg press, chest press, jogging.
Slow twitch – endurance fibres Slow to contract, slow to tire Preference for continuous activity, fatigue resistant Work at lower intensities (30% of maximal contraction)	Fast twitch – strength fibres Quick to contract, quick to tire Preference for more intense activity, fatigue quicker Work at higher intensities (higher % of maximal contraction)
Recruited at between 20-30% of voluntary contraction	Recruited above 40% of voluntary contraction
Tendency to lengthen and become inactive	Tendency to shorten and become overactive/tight
Work on shortening muscles within inner range Increase activity	Work on lengthening (static or PNF stretching) reduces dependency on them

Adapted from Northern Fitness and Education, *Modern Pilates Stage One* (2004a)

Progressing muscular fitness exercises

There are five specific methods for adapting and progressing the intensity of muscular fitness exercises. These are:

- Repetitions
- Rest (between sets or exercises)
- Range of motion
- Rate/speed
- Resistance

Repetitions, rest and sets

The ACSM (2005) recommends a broad range of repetitions (between 3 and 20). The number of repetitions (and sets, or repeats of an exercise) can be increased or decreased to meet different fitness goals (strength or endurance). Repetitions can initially be low and then be progressively increased, moving from developing strength to enhancing endurance.

For some individuals, as few as 1 to 3 repetitions of an exercise would be an appropriate starting point to develop activity and strength of the muscle and to perform the exercise with correct alignment and technique. The muscle can then be rested for a short time by resting completely (doing nothing), working another muscle or stretching the muscle worked. If further challenge is required, another set of that exercise could be performed. Progression can be achieved by reducing the duration of the rest time between sets.

Rate

Exercise should always be performed at a controlled speed to promote full range of motion of concentric and eccentric muscle work.

Varying the speed of an exercise will alter the intensity and may also change the focus on the muscle contraction. For example, varying the

speed to work faster on the lifting phase and slower on the lowering phase will focus on the eccentric contraction range. Caution is advised when lengthening the eccentric phase, as this may cause delayed onset muscle soreness (ACSM 2005).

In Pilates, movements are generally performed at a slower pace to maintain the control needed and connect the movements and breathing. However, different schools do emphasise different ways of working with speed.

The recommendation of integrated Pilates would be to be flexible and adaptable, consider the needs of the individual(s) and allow individuals to work at a speed that suits their skill, ability and training goals.

For example, when performing a shoulder bridge:

The movement could initially be performed slower (and even through a smaller range of motion);

There could be a short hold at the top to regain the control needed to roll down sequentially;

There could be a longer hold at the top (even adding another movement of the arms or legs) to challenge stability before rolling down;

The movement could flow, rolling up and rolling down without pauses.

Range of motion

It is generally recommended that muscle work occur though the full range of motion. However, there are some instances where isometric and static muscle work are more beneficial as a starting point, for example training core stability and posture and for some joint mobility problems (osteoarthritis).

The range of motion can be gradually increased in certain exercises to provide progression. For example:

A shoulder bridge can initially be performed

as a pelvic tilt;

Arm raises and floats can be performed through a smaller range of motion by lifting a smaller distance;

Standing knee raises can initially be performed as a heel raise.

Resistance

There are numerous methods for altering the resistance within a Pilates session, such as:

- Increasing (or decreasing) the length of the lever being moved. Shorter levers are easier to move than longer levers.
- Adding (or removing) weight to/from the exercise. This might be body weight or external equipment such as weight/exercise bands, circles and balls.
- Working against (or working across) gravity.
- Progressing to train and work with specialised Pilates equipment.

Motor fitness

Motor fitness is a skill-related component of fitness and refers to a number of inter-relatable factors, which include:

- Agility
- Balance
- Speed
- Co-ordination
- Reaction time
- Power

Benefits of motor fitness

Motor fitness requires the effective transmission and management of messages and responses between the central nervous system or CNS (the brain and spinal cord) and the peripheral nervous system (sensory and motor). The peripheral system collects information via the sensory system. The CNS receives and processes this information and sends an appropriate response via the motor system, which initiates the appropriate response.

Motor fitness can have an indirect effect on improving our ability to function in the other components of fitness. Development of specific motor skills can improve our performance of certain activities and enable more skilful movement and safer exercise techniques. This can help to reduce the risk of injury and will maximise both the safety and effectiveness of performance.

Motor fitness applied to the Pilates method

Exercises that require maintenance of correct posture, transference of the body weight, movement changes of the centre of gravity, co-ordination of combined body movements (arms and legs), in different directions and at different speeds will all contribute to developing motor fitness within a Pilates session.

Skilful and controlled movement is an integral component of the Pilates method. Learning to balance, co-ordinate and develop stability to perform movement patterns safely and effectively takes time and practice. It is essential to start with the simplest movements and progress gradually. In addition, breaking down the more complex movement patterns and exercises into their simpler alternatives can enable progressive learning and skill development.

Relearning movement patterns takes equal time. As a general guideline, starting slower, with isolated movements, simpler movement patterns and focusing on correct performance of these movements helps to provide the foundation for developing motor fitness. Patience, encouragement and raising awareness to small changes and progression are essential to maintain motivation.

Developing motor fitness with the Pilates method

Here are some guidelines and considerations for developing motor fitness with the Pilates method:

- Develop the basic principles first (ABC).
- Learn to perform and maintain the correct start positions – standing, seated, hands and knees, prone lying, supine and supine crook (lying on back with legs straight and legs bent respectively), side lying and kneeling.

- Start with the most stable and functional positions (supine lying, standing and seated) and develop to positions where the base of support is less stable (side lying, hands and knees, or using stability equipment such as balls and boards).
- Initially perform simple and isolated movements from start positions and progress to combining movements.
- Start with shorter leverage (less weight), smaller range of movement and slower speed and progressively develop these principles to challenge stability, mobility and skill development.
- Increase repetitions progressively when correct patterns of movement have been learned with positive reinforcement.

TOTAL FITNESS AND THE PILATES METHOD

3

Total fitness provides a model from which assessments regarding an individual's overall health and well-being can be monitored. It requires balanced 'fitness' in all the following areas:

Physically

Achieving recommended levels of physical activity in daily lifestyle and taking part in exercise to maintain physical fitness in the components discussed in the previous chapter.

Socially

Being able to create and maintain healthy relationships with others and with society.

Mentally

Having an awareness of personal thinking patterns and being able to manage thinking to assist positive decision making and life choices.

Emotionally

Having an awareness of emotions (such as happiness, sadness, fear, anger), and the ability to manage and express them assertively with respect for oneself and others.

Nutritionally

Eating a balanced diet containing a variety of foods from all major food groups (carbohydrates, fats, protein, vitamins, minerals, water, fibre), eaten within recommended guidelines and maintaining a balanced calorific intake to meet energy demands.

Medically

Being free from illness and disease and making positive life choices to maintain medical health.

Spiritually

Having an awareness of one's belief systems, which may evolve from one's family, society, culture and religion, and managing these to make positive decisions for oneself and others, embracing the notions of difference and similarity among people.

Social fitness

Social fitness relates to interaction and communication with other people, and the ability to form and maintain healthy functional relationships within society.

The physical changes that can occur from regular Pilates practice (improved posture, muscle tone, mobility and body shape) may increase the individual's confidence to reach out and make friends. Psychological wellness may improve (increased feelings of competence and esteem) as the individual masters specific activities and receives praise and encouragement.

As a group exercise, Pilates offers an opportunity to meet people with a common interest and as a consequence friendships and other social opportunities may develop.

Mental and emotional fitness

Mental and emotional fitness refer to psychological well-being. The pressures of daily life (physical, mental, emotional) can have a negative effect on our mental and emotional well-being and these stresses can sometimes be observed in the body. Lack of confidence and self-esteem may contribute to a person rounding their posture forwards and looking down at the floor as they walk. This in turn may affect their muscle balance and cause postural misalignment (kyphosis).

Stress can also create muscular tension, a consequence of the body preparing for 'fight or flight' without the actual physical release.

Pilates has a specific focus on relaxation and concentration that can be used to assist with managing the stress response and improving mental and emotional well-being. Firstly, the slower and more controlled nature of the movements offer a contrast to the more hurried way in which many of us operate on a daily basis. The focus on breathing and use of the breath offers a distraction by focusing the mind away from external stressors and on to the body and the self. Slowing down one's breathing also helps slow down other bodily systems that are triggered by stress. Stretching within the sessions will lengthen muscles that have become shortened. The focus on mobility can unknot tension in muscles, allowing freedom of movement to be regained. These are a few of the many benefits.

Nutritional fitness

Nutritional fitness requires us to eat a balanced diet of foods from all the major food groups in the appropriate quantities to maintain nutritional and energy requirements. The foods we eat will affect how much energy we have, as well as our health and well-being. There are no bad foods per se, just poor diets.

The main food groups are:

- Carbohydrates (pasta, potatoes, bread)
- Fats (cheese, milk, butter)
- Proteins (beans, pulses, meat)
- Vitamins and minerals (vegetables and fruit)
- Water

Taking part in regular physical activity can make us more conscious of our diet. There are many books devoted to nutrition; some of these are listed at the end of this book. Some general guidelines for improving our diet are:

- Eat less saturated fat. Too much increases the risk of high cholesterol and furring of the artery walls.
- Eat less sugar. Too much can cause tooth decay and contribute to us being overweight or obese.
- Eat less salt. Too much may elevate blood pressure.
- Eat more complex carbohydrates. Too little will lower our energy levels.
- Eat sufficient fibre. Too little may cause constipation and other bowel disorders.
- Eat more fruit and vegetables (five portions a day).
- Take in the right amount of calories. Too few will slow down our metabolism and make us feel lethargic; too many will make us put on weight and will be stored as body fat.
- Drink more water. Too little fluid will cause dehydration, potential heat stroke and place an unnecessary stress on the heart.
- Eat when you feel hungry. If we do not eat when we feel hungry our blood sugar levels will be affected, causing us to overeat and/or eat the wrong type of foods to manage our sugar levels. In addition, some people confuse hunger with other feelings or emotional

experiences and can use food to comfort them. Eating more than we need for energy will contribute to us being overweight or obese.

Spiritual fitness

Spirituality for me embraces the concept of finding harmony and balance within and between our inner world (thoughts, feelings and so on) and our outer worlds (work, relationships, materialism).

For many people, and for most of life, a lot more focus is given to the outer world and developing success in this area than to looking inwards and being successful there. It is often the case that the only time we are stretched to look within is during critical life events such as illness and experience of death or loss. These events can trigger and awaken the existential search to find answers for being, and can provide an opportunity for spiritual growth, which is a lifelong journey! However, as Van Deurzen (2000:333) suggests: 'Some people manage to overcome substantial initial disadvantages or adversity, whereas others squander their advantage or flounder in the face of minor contretemps.'

From a spiritual perspective, each of us is a unique individual with our own life journey and our own life lessons. We each make choices to follow our life path (whether conscious or unconscious) and we each have the potential and inner power to choose how we respond to, and grow from, life's challenges.

The principles of awareness, breathing and alignment, which we discussed in chapter 1, can help us learn to engage with the self on a physical, mental, emotional and spiritual level.

Medical fitness

Medical fitness is our state of health. It requires the body to be in optimal working order.

Pilates focuses on training components of physical fitness that can contribute to improving and managing a number of muscular and skeletal conditions, including low back pain, osteoporosis, osteoarthritis and postural conditions (discussed in chapter 7). It can also assist with managing stress and developing better patterns of breathing (see chapter 8). The latter can assist with management of respiratory conditions such as COPD and asthma.

Summary of the potential health and total fitness benefits of Pilates

- Improve posture and ease of movement
- Maintain and improve mobility and flexibility
- Improve strength of bones and muscles
- Improve strength and endurance of the core muscles and promote greater stability
- Improve breathing and assist management of respiratory conditions
- Encourage a healthier lifestyle
- Improve sleep patterns and increase energy levels
- Improve self-esteem and confidence
- Manage joint and mobility conditions
- Improve ability to carry out everyday activities and help maintain independence
- Assist with managing activity of the mind and emotions.

ANATOMY APPLIED TO THE PILATES METHOD

Part two introduces and focuses on some of the skeletal structures and their muscular attachments that are applicable to the Pilates method. It is assumed that readers will have a basic knowledge of anatomy and physiology, equivalent to Level 2 of the National Occupational Standards (NOS).

If you are interested in reading further and extending your knowledge in these areas, the references mention useful books, in particular *Anatomy of Hatha Yoga* by H. David Coulter.

The major muscles – anterior view

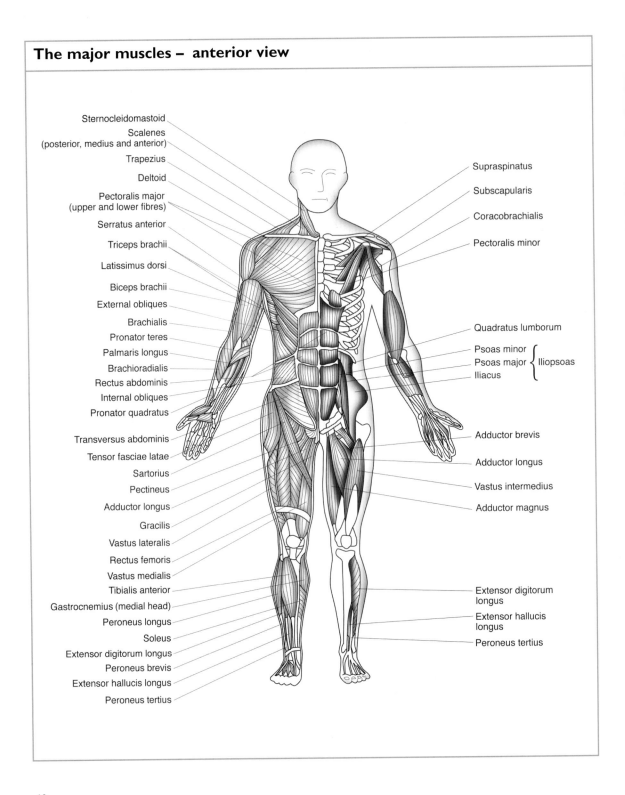

Sternocleidomastoid
Scalenes
(posterior, medius and anterior)
Trapezius
Deltoid
Pectoralis major
(upper and lower fibres)
Serratus anterior
Triceps brachii
Latissimus dorsi
Biceps brachii
External obliques
Brachialis
Pronator teres
Palmaris longus
Brachioradialis
Rectus abdominis
Internal obliques
Pronator quadratus
Transversus abdominis
Tensor fasciae latae
Sartorius
Pectineus
Adductor longus
Gracilis
Vastus lateralis
Rectus femoris
Vastus medialis
Tibialis anterior
Gastrocnemius (medial head)
Peroneus longus
Soleus
Extensor digitorum longus
Peroneus brevis
Extensor hallucis longus
Peroneus tertius

Supraspinatus
Subscapularis
Coracobrachialis
Pectoralis minor
Quadratus lumborum
Psoas minor
Psoas major   } Iliopsoas
Iliacus
Adductor brevis
Adductor longus
Vastus intermedius
Adductor magnus
Extensor digitorum longus
Extensor hallucis longus
Peroneus tertius

The major muscles – posterior view

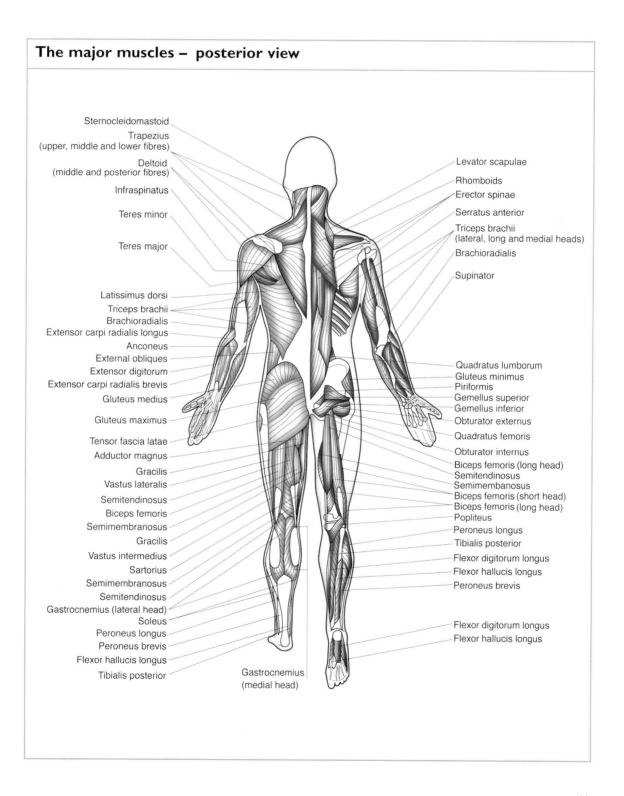

Sternocleidomastoid
Trapezius
(upper, middle and lower fibres)
Deltoid
(middle and posterior fibres)
Infraspinatus
Teres minor
Teres major

Latissimus dorsi
Triceps brachii
Brachioradialis
Extensor carpi radialis longus
Anconeus
External obliques
Extensor digitorum
Extensor carpi radialis brevis
Gluteus medius
Gluteus maximus
Tensor fascia latae
Adductor magnus
Gracilis
Vastus lateralis
Semitendinosus
Biceps femoris
Semimembranosus
Gracilis
Vastus intermedius
Sartorius
Semimembranosus
Semitendinosus
Gastrocnemius (lateral head)
Soleus
Peroneus longus
Peroneus brevis
Flexor hallucis longus
Tibialis posterior

Gastrocnemius
(medial head)

Levator scapulae
Rhomboids
Erector spinae
Serratus anterior
Triceps brachii
(lateral, long and medial heads)
Brachioradialis

Supinator

Quadratus lumborum
Gluteus minimus
Piriformis
Gemellus superior
Gemellus inferior
Obturator externus
Quadratus femoris

Obturator internus
Biceps femoris (long head)
Semitendinosus
Semimembranosus
Biceps femoris (short head)
Biceps femoris (long head)
Popliteus
Peroneus longus
Tibialis posterior
Flexor digitorum longus
Flexor hallucis longus
Peroneus brevis

Flexor digitorum longus
Flexor hallucis longus

The major bones

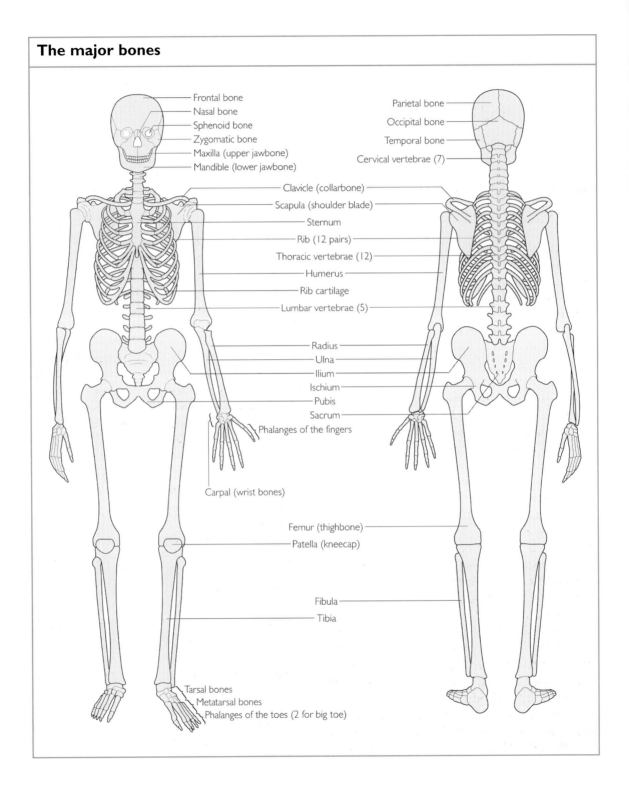

Frontal bone
Nasal bone
Sphenoid bone
Zygomatic bone
Maxilla (upper jawbone)
Mandible (lower jawbone)

Parietal bone
Occipital bone
Temporal bone
Cervical vertebrae (7)

Clavicle (collarbone)
Scapula (shoulder blade)
Sternum
Rib (12 pairs)
Thoracic vertebrae (12)
Humerus
Rib cartilage
Lumbar vertebrae (5)

Radius
Ulna
Ilium
Ischium
Pubis
Sacrum
Phalanges of the fingers

Carpal (wrist bones)

Femur (thighbone)
Patella (kneecap)

Fibula
Tibia

Tarsal bones
Metatarsal bones
Phalanges of the toes (2 for big toe)

THE SPINE

4

Structure of the vertebral column

The vertebral column, or spine, forms part of the *axial skeleton.* It extends from the base of the skull to the bottom of the pelvis and measures between 70 and 75cm in the average adult.

The spine is composed of a series of 33 irregular bones called *vertebrae*, which progressively increase in size, being smaller at the top and larger at the bottom of the spine. The 24 superior (upper) bones present as individual bones to form the cervical, thoracic and lumbar sections of the spine. The inferior (lower) nine vertebrae are fused – joined together (before adulthood) to form the sacrum and coccyx.

In between each of the individual bones there are cartilage discs. These *intervertebral discs* give the spine its flexibility and movement, and also assist with absorbing some of the impact stress that is transmitted through the body. The intervertebral discs also provide approximately a quarter of the spine's length. Thinning of these discs can account for changes in height among older adults. In addition, changes in disc compressibility throughout the day can account for other minor changes in height measurement. For example, when the spine is rested (after a long sleep) and the discs are hydrated, the individual may be slightly taller than when the spine has been carrying the body weight during daily activities and the discs are dehydrated. This may have an effect on postural assessment. Therefore, to maximise accuracy of information gathered, it is recommended that postural assessments be made at the same time of day and in similar conditions.

The spine has natural curvatures provided by the rounding and hollowing of its different regions. These curvatures give the spine its characteristic S shape, which further increases the spine's capacity to absorb impact without injury. The degree of curvature in the spine can vary between individuals, sometimes due to genetics but sometimes because of poor posture or muscle tone or imbalance in the supporting muscles. Posture, posture types and factors affecting posture are discussed further in chapter 7.

The vertebrae in the neck are called the *cervical* vertebrae. There are seven in total. This region of the spine has a concave or hollow curvature.

The vertebrae of the trunk or thorax are called the *thoracic* vertebrae. There are 12 in total. This region of the spine has a convex or rounded curvature.

The vertebrae of the lower back are called the *lumbar* vertebrae. There are five in total. This region of the spine has a concave or hollow curvature.

The vertebrae that join with the iliac bones to form the pelvis are called the *sacral* vertebrae (sacrum). There are five in total and they are fused together. This region of the spine has a convex or rounded curvature.

The vertebrae that form the tailbone or coccyx are called the *coccygeal* vertebrae. There are four of these tiny bones and they are fused.

Fig. 4.1	The spine

Cervical vertebrae (×7)

Thoracic vertebrae (×12)

Invertebral discs

Invertebral foramina

Lumbar vertebrae (×5)

Sacrum (×5)

Coccyx (2–4)

Functions of the vertebral column

Palastanga et al (1989) identify a number of functions of the vertebral column. These include:

- Support for the head/skull
- Support and point of attachment for the thoracic cage (ribcage)
- Attachment point for muscles of the shoulder and pelvic girdle
- Attachment point for muscles that mobilise and maintain stability and erectness of the vertebral column (spine extensors and flexors)
- Encloses and provides protection (via the vertebral foramina) for the spinal cord
- Shock absorption from impact when the body is moving (intervertebral discs and natural curvatures)
- Movement via the different vertebral sections.

Structure of the vertebrae

There are variations in the size and shape of the vertebrae in different areas of the spine. However, most individual vertebrae have a number of common features:

A bony body

At the front (anterior) there is a large disc-shaped bony body that forms the weight-bearing aspect of the vertebrae.

Intervertebral discs

Cartilage discs are positioned above and below (superior and inferior) the bony body, connecting each of the vertebrae together. The discs assist with cushioning some of the impact forces through the spine. Damage to the fibrous outer ring of the intervertebral discs can allow some of the gel-like interior to extrude. This may result in compression of one of the spinal nerves, causing intense pain and potential paralysis in muscles supplied by the compressed nerve.

A vertebral arch

At the rear (posterior) of the vertebrae is the vertebral or neural arch. The vertebral arch is the opposite side of the bony body (the vertebral canal is the centre of these two structures). It is composed of two bony processes (pedicles and lamina). The pedicles project from the back (posterior) of the bony body and join with the lamina (at both sides), to form the vertebral arch.

Processes

A number of spinous processes arise from the vertebral arch. The transverse process extends at both sides (laterally) where the pedicles and lamina meet, and a spinous process extends from the rear (posterior) and slightly below (inferiorly) to the lamina. These function as an attachment point for the muscles of the back. The other four processes (the two superior articular processes and the two inferior articular processes) articulate with adjacent vertebrae (above and below respectively) to form *facet joints*. These gliding synovial joints are covered with hyaline cartilage to provide movement. The position of the facet joints in different regions of the spine largely determines the degree of movement available in each section of the spine. This is discussed further in the following pages.

A vertebral foramen

At the centre of each vertebra between the anterior body and posterior arch is an opening (vertebral foramina), which provides a protective channel for the *spinal cord*. The spinal

---

Fig. 4.2   Atlas and Axis (a) superior view (b) anterior view

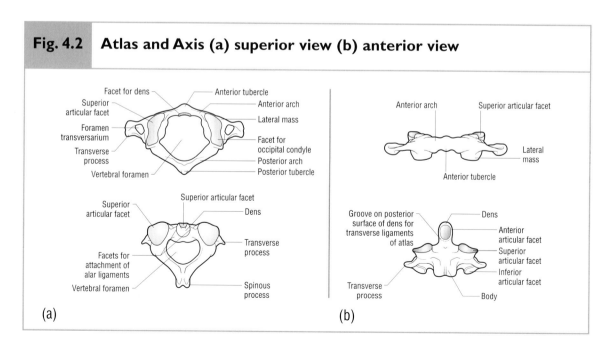

(a)   (b)

nerves exit the vertebral column through small spaces in between the processes.

Ligaments

Ligaments stretch along the length of the vertebral column, attaching bone to bone at the front (anteriorly) and at the back (posteriorly). They provide the support needed to keep the column erect. The anterior ligaments are broader and comparatively stronger; they attach both to the bones and the intervertebral discs. The posterior ligaments are narrower and comparatively weak. This makes them more susceptible to damage when bending forwards quickly. There are also many short ligaments that connect each vertebra to the one just above and below it. Again, these are relatively weak and may be damaged with excessive movement.

The vertebrae in each of the different regions also have special characteristics, which allow them to perform more specialised functions and movements.

Cervical vertebrae

The cervical vertebrae (C1 to C7) are the smallest of the vertebrae. They are not designed to carry weight and are susceptible to injury if moved too quickly.

The *atlas* is the first of the cervical vertebrae (C1). It is positioned at the top of the spine and is essentially a bony ring on which the skull rests and balances. It shares little resemblance in appearance to other vertebrae, in that it has no main body or spiny process (see Fig. 4.2).

The synovial joint that occurs between the atlas and the skull allows forward and backward nodding movements – *flexion and extension* – and also side bending movements – *lateral flexion and lateral extension.*

The *axis* is the second and strongest of the

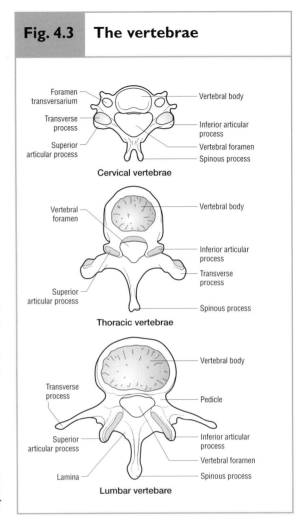

Fig. 4.3   The vertebrae

Cervical vertebrae

Thoracic vertebrae

Lumbar vertebare

cervical vertebra (C2). It has a rounded, peg-like projection called the odontoid process (dens), which projects upwards into the ring of the atlas to form a synovial pivot joint that allows twisting movements of the neck or *rotation* (see Fig. 4.2).

The facet joints in the upper region of the cervical vertebrae are positioned at a slightly backward angle and allow considerable movement in all planes.

The lower cervical vertebrae (C3 to C6) are more uniform and oval-shaped in appearance.

In the lower regions of the cervical vertebrae, the facets become more vertical. Movement available in the lower cervical vertebrae is therefore limited.

The lowest cervical vertebrae is the *vertebra prominens* (C7). It is larger than the other vertebrae and has a much longer spinous process (hence the name). This spinous process can be felt at the base of the neck.

Thoracic vertebrae

The thoracic vertebrae (T1 to T12) are larger and stronger than the cervical vertebrae. They have heart-shaped bony bodies and a longer spinous process that is directed downwards (inferiorly) to the rear (posterior). They have two facets at each side. One facet articulates with the ribs (the exceptions being T11 and T12); the other articulates with the adjacent vertebrae.

The attachment of the thoracic vertebrae to the ribs assists spine mobility. Lateral breathing exercises that encourage the ribcage to move three-dimensionally – to the front, side and back – can help increase mobility in the thoracic region.

The facet joints in the thoracic vertebrae are positioned more vertically. Therefore, individually, each vertebra has a very small range of movement. However, the number of vertebrae in the thoracic area is greater than the number in other regions of the spine. For this reason, the thoracic region is the most movable area of the spine, allowing flexion and extension, lateral flexion and extension and some degree of rotation.

Lumbar vertebrae

The lumbar vertebrae (L1 to L5) are the largest and strongest of the vertebrae. They have large, sturdy kidney-shaped bony bodies and thick intervertebral discs. The spinous processes in this area of the spine are wider and thicker and project almost straight to the rear (posteriorly). The facet joints are positioned so that the five vertebrae are almost locked together, restricting the amount of twisting or rotation that can occur. Movements that attempt to rotate the lumbar vertebrae can cause damage to the facet joints and may decrease the stability of the whole vertebral column.

The lumbar vertebrae can safely perform forward bending, or flexion (a total range of 55 degrees) and backward bending, or extension (a total range of 30 degrees). Less movement is available at the thoracolumbar junction (the upper region) and more movement is available at the lumbo-sacral joint, the lower region (where L5 meets S1). The lumbar spine can also perform side bending, or lateral flexion and extension (a total range between 30 and 60 degrees). The total range of movement available decreases with age.

Care must be taken when performing movements of the spine to ensure maximal control within a safe range of movement (this will vary between individuals) in order to minimise compression of the intervertebral discs. Excessive movements of the spine, hyperflexion and hyperextension, should therefore be performed with great care. For some individuals, they should be avoided so as not to cause injury to the discs.

The lumbar vertebrae cope with most of the impact stress that occurs during movement and activities that involve jumping and running. Correct alignment is therefore essential. In addition, the lumbar or lordotic curve has a critical role to play in spinal stability and should be neither too flat (flat back) nor too hollow (lordotic) – for more information, see chapter 7 on posture and posture types. Instead a 'neutral spine' position should be encouraged. The neutral spine/pelvic position is described in chapter 1.

Sacrum

The sacrum is a triangular shape and is formed by the fusion of the five sacral vertebrae (S1 to S5). It provides a strong foundation for the pelvic girdle and is joined at each side (laterally) with the right and left iliac bones (ilium) to provide the sacroiliac joint. Further information on the pelvic girdle is provided in chapter 5.

Coccyx

The coccyx, or tail bone, is also triangular in shape and is formed by the joining of the second to fourth coccygeal vertebrae. The top (superior) aspect of the coccyx joins with the sacrum. The coccyx can be damaged when falling backwards and landing on the bottom.

Fig. 4.4	**Curvatures of the spine**

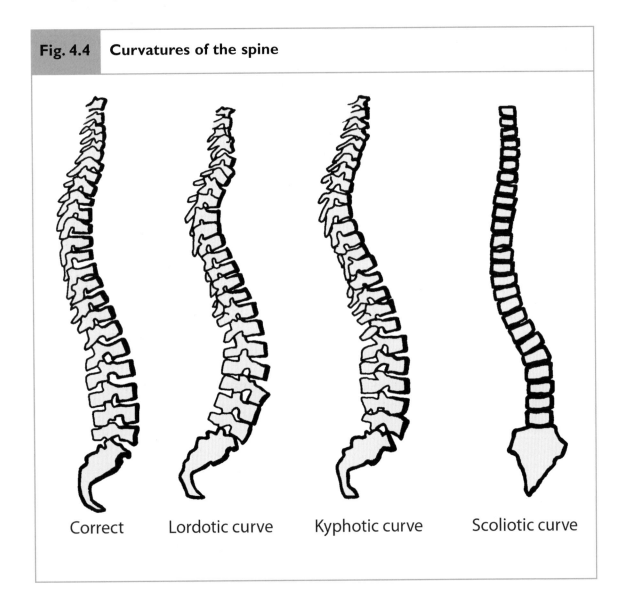

Correct   Lordotic curve   Kyphotic curve   Scoliotic curve

Muscles supporting the vertebral column

There are a number of muscles that support the vertebral column to the front (anterior), sides (lateral) and back (posterior). These muscles

Table 4.1	Erector spinae	
Iliocostalis lumborum	Longissimus thoracis	
Iliocostalis thoracis	Longissimus cervicis	
Iliocostalis cervicis	Longissimus capitis	
Spinalis thoracis	Spinalis cervicis	
Description and muscle action	Closer to the body surface (superficial) Positioned at the rear/posterior Run down the length of the whole vertebral column	
Actions:	• Extension of vertebral column • Lateral flexion of vertebral column • Rotates ribs for forceful expiration • Stabilises the spine when dead- lifting a weight from floor to thigh level • Stabilises the spine during squatting movements (bending the knees and hips)	

Table 4.2	Multifidus
Needs to be strong to counteract the pull of the hip flexor on the lumbar spine (which will pull the spine into hyperextension) during hip flexion movements.	
Description and muscle action	Deeper than the erector spinae group Runs down the length of the spine Positioned in the space between the transverse and spinous processes of the vertebrae Spans and joins between one and three vertebral sections
Actions:	Both sides working together (bilateral) • Extends vertebral column • Keeps the spine stable (stiff) during lifting of resistance) • Key functional role as a stabiliser muscle Each side working in isolation (unilateral) • Rotation of spine (Stone & Stone, 1990)

Table 4.3	Quadratus Lumborum
Description and muscle action	Positioned at the side and back of the body Deeper than the erector spinae group Attaches from the top of the iliac crest (right and left sides) to the twelfth rib and transverse processes of the lumbar vertebrae (L1 to L4) Is enclosed by the front (anterior) and middle layers of the thoracolumbar fascia
Actions:	Both sides working together (bilateral) • Assists erector spinae in extension of the spine • Fixes the twelfth ribs during deep inspiration (Stone & Stone, 1990) Each side working alone in isolation (unilateral) • Working concentrically, brings about lateral flexion • Working eccentrically, helps prevent hyperflexion laterally (to opposite side) • Keeps the spine stable when carrying heavy loads in one hand (Thompson, 1989) When standing on one leg, acts strongly to prevent the pelvis dropping on the weight-bearing leg

work together to maintain correct posture and alignment of the vertebral column or spine. Any imbalance in the strength and flexibility of these muscles can result in incorrect alignment of the spine and may contribute to postural misalignment and curvatures.

An imbalance between the strength and flexibility of the muscles that flex the spine (abdominals) and the opposite muscles that extend the spine (back muscles) can contribute to an exaggerated curve or hollowing of the lumbar vertebrae (lordosis). An imbalance of strength and flexibility between the muscles of the chest (the pectorals) and the muscles between the shoulder blades (the rhomboids and trapezius) can cause rounded shoulders and a humping of the thoracic spine (kyphosis). An imbalance in strength between the muscles on each side of the back can cause a sideways curvature of the thoracic spine (scoliosis).

All muscles should therefore be kept sufficiently strong and flexible to maintain a correct alignment of the vertebral column. Posture types are discussed further in chapter 7.

Muscles supporting the spine at the back and sides

Note: Refer to the major muscles diagrams on pp. 40–41 for the position of the different muscles.

Thoracolumbar fascia (TLF)

This is a diamond-shaped fascia (tendon) positioned in the lower back (posterior) region of the body, between the pelvis and the thoracic spine. A number of muscles are connected on to the thoracolumbar fascia (transversus abdominis, internal obliques, quadratus lumborum, erector spinae, latissimus dorsi, gluteus maximus).

When these muscles contract, they pull on the fascia, providing a tightening effect that helps maintain the stability of the spine and prevent the spine collapsing into a flexed or bent forward position. All of the muscles that connect to the TLF will help to keep it taut, thereby keeping a firmness to the back wall of what is sometimes referred to by Norris (2001) as the abdominal balloon or inner core unit.

The fascia consists of three layers that are positioned progressively deeper in the body – a posterior (most superficial, back) layer, a middle layer and an anterior (deepest, front) layer. The posterior layer is more superficial to erector spinae and spans from the pelvis (iliac crest and sacrum) to the vertebrae and angles of the ribs. Latissimus dorsi arises from the lower portion. The middle layer is sandwiched between erector spinae and the deeper quadratus lumborum. The anterior layer lies in front of (anterior to) quadratus lumborum. The internal obliques and transversus abdominis attach to the sides (lateral) of this fascia.

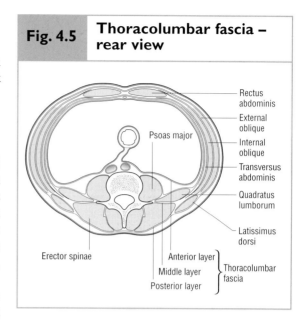

Fig. 4.5 Thoracolumbar fascia – rear view

Rectus abdominis
External oblique
Psoas major
Internal oblique
Transversus abdominis
Quadratus lumborum
Latissimus dorsi
Erector spinae
Anterior layer
Middle layer
Posterior layer
Thoracolumbar fascia

Muscles supporting the spine from the front and side

Note: Refer to The major muscles diagrams on pp. 40–41 for the position of the different muscles.

The abdominal muscles provide the anterior (front) support to the vertebral column. The abdominals consist of three layers of flat, broad muscles that have fibres running at different angles to each other.

Fig. 4.6	The abdominal muscles

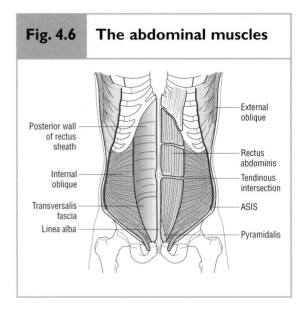

Table 4.4	Rectus abdominis
Description and muscle action	Two strips of superficially positioned muscle with vertically aligned straight fibres attaching from the pubis symphysis (both sides) to the cartilage of the lower fifth to seventh ribs (both sides) and the bottom of the sternum or breastbone. Each side divides into four sections with tendonous inscriptions between each section. This provides the 'six pack' look for lean and muscular individuals. The muscles are separated centrally and join with other abdominal muscles at the linea alba, a fibrous band running down the centre of the body from the base of the sternum (breastbone) to the pubis symphysis.
Actions:	• Flexion of spine • Lateral flexion of spine (Thompson, 1989) • Compresses abdomen (Stone and Stone, 1990)

Table 4.5	External obliques
Description and muscle action	Superficially positioned broad band of muscle at each side of the trunk with downward and inward slanted or oblique fibres. Attaches from the lower eight ribs to the front of the pelvis (iliac crest) and forms an aponeurosis (muscle attaching to other muscles) at the linea alba.
Actions:	Working together (bilateral) • Flexion of spine (Thompson, 1989) • Compression of the abdomen (Stone & Stone, 1989) Working alone (unilateral) • Rotation of spine (right side twists to left and left side twists to right – Thompson, 1989) • Lateral flexion of spine (Stone & Stone, 1990)

Table 4.6	Internal obliques
Description and muscle action	Broad band of muscle running underneath external obliques at both sides of the body with slanted or oblique fibres running upwards and inwards. Attaches from thoracolumbar fascia, pelvis (iliac crest) and inguinal ligament to the cartilage of lower three to four ribs.
Actions:	Working together (bilateral) • Assists with flexion of spine • Compresses abdomen (Stone & Stone, 1990) Working alone (unilateral) • Rotation of spine (right side of muscle twists to right and left side of muscle twists to left – Thompson, 1989) • Lateral flexion of spine

Table 4.7	Transversus abdominis
Description and muscle action	Deepest layer of muscle in the abdominal wall, with fibres running horizontally around the trunk to form a corset. Attaches from the linea alba to the inguinal ligament, pelvis (iliac crest) and cartilage of lower six ribs.
Actions:	• Compresses the abdomen (Stone & Stone, 1990) and gives a flatter appearance to the abdominal area • Supports the abdominal contents • Forced expiration – pulls the abdominal wall inward (Thompson, 1989)

Theory into practice – application

The core muscles are those that form what Norris (2001) refers to as a 'cylinder' that creates the 'abdominal balloon' effect. They include:

- Transversus abdominis, which forms a corset around the centre (anterior – front wall).
- Internal obliques and quadratus lumborum (lateral – side wall).
- Multifidus and the thoracolumbar fascia (posterior – back wall).
- The diaphragm, the main breathing muscle, forming the top of the cylinder (superior – top wall). Breathing will be discussed further in chapter 8.
- The pelvic floor, forming the bottom seal of the cylinder (inferior – lower wall). The pelvic floor will be discussed further in chapter 5.

During larger movements of the spine in all the different movement planes (curl-ups, back raises, side bends and so on), the superficial muscles (rectus abdominis, erector spinae and external obliques) are most active. In addition,

our lack of attention to, and awareness of, movement means that we tend to overuse these muscles.

The deeper 'core' muscles (transversus abdominis, quadratus lumborum, multifidus, internal obliques) also need to be strong to prevent unnecessary movements of the vertebrae during the aforementioned movements. They also need to be engaged and strong when we are lifting heavy objects to maintain the neutral position of the spine/pelvis described in chapter 1. If these muscles are not sufficiently strong, there is a danger that the neutral position is lost and alignment will be compromised.

The abdominal balloon in action

When all the core muscles work in synchrony, the 'inner cylinder' is squeezed from all directions (top, bottom, sides, front and back). This squeezing builds up pressure in the abdominal cavity. 'Intra-abdominal pressure' creates a strong foundation in the trunk so that the spine is kept stable and aligned. It could be visualised as like having an 'air bag' or 'bubble' (Norris, 2001) inside protecting the spine.

However, developing synchronicity between contraction of each wall of the cylinder is where the system can break down. Weakness in any area will impair the effectiveness of this cylinder. For example: an overweight/obese and/or sedentary person, or an individual with untrained abdominals, may have poor muscle tone and lengthened abdominal muscles. Some older adults and new mothers may have weakened pelvic floor muscles. Persons with back problems or who have undergone surgery in this region will be weaker in this area. Thus, the aim of the Pilates method is to redevelop this synchronicity and balance.

In addition to this, the core muscles also pull against the thoracolumbar fascia from different angles, which creates a tightening effect around the mid section and pulls the fascia tight. Baker (2004) describes as 'a bit like pulling on the back of a shirt' (Northern Fitness and Education, 2004).

During performance of the following exercises, individuals should be encouraged to engage the core muscles (25-30 per cent of maximal contraction) from a position of optimal posture and alignment (correct start position) and work towards sustaining the contraction during exercises performed from this start position. The engagement of the abdominals should also be co-ordinated with the breath:

Breathing in to prepare for the movement;

Breathing out and engaging the core to move (the effort – usually lifting – phase);

Breathe in (maintain abdominal engagement) on the return to the start position (this is usually the lowering phase).

Another key point to consider when training the core stabilisers is to ensure minimal activity of the hip flexor muscles!

Modified exercises

Exercise 4.1 Seated spine rotation/twist (all levels)

See Ex. 4.1

Purpose

- Spine mobility – rotation
- Pelvic stability
- Scapular stability and ribcage placement isolation and control
- Endurance for oblique muscles

Start position

Seated (floor or block)

Place hands in line with shoulders at the side of body and should maintain alignment with shoulders throughout. Visualise fingers moving through a pool of water.

Instructions and teaching points

1. Inhale to prepare.
2. Exhale, engage abdominals and lift out of the hip, extending the spine (visualise head being lifted upwards to the ceiling).
3. Rotate to one side, focus on sequentially turning each vertebra from the waist upwards and imagine twisting around a broom handle placed along length of spine (floor to ceiling).
4. Inhale to return.

Variations

- Hand can be placed in prayer position in front of the breastbone, ensuring shoulder girdle slides down.
- Hands can be held in a W position (arms at shoulder height, elbows bent at 90 degrees with hands facing forwards and fingers pointing towards ceiling). Take care as this will contract deltoids isometrically and may cause shoulders to elevate.
- Seated on a block for persons unable to sit upright on sitting bones
- Chair seated
- Standing

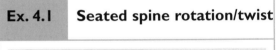

Ex. 4.1   Seated spine rotation/twist

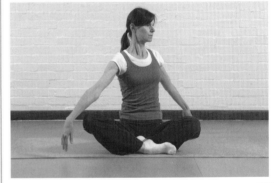

Exercise 4.2 Supine pelvic tilt

See Ex. 4.2

Ex. 4.2   Supine pelvic tilt

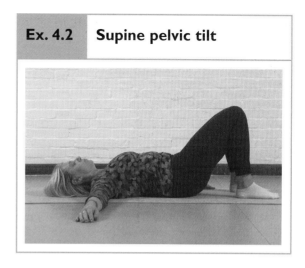

Purpose

- Lumbar spine mobility – lumbar flexion and extension
- Strengthen abdominals, gluteals, abductors
- Pelvic stability

Start position

Supine crook lying

Use towel or block under head to ensure correct alignment of neck

Instructions and teaching points

1. Inhale to prepare.
2. Exhale, engage abdominals, tilt pelvis so that back flattens towards floor and engage gluteals.
3. Inhale to lower and sequentially roll back to neutral.
4. Keep shoulders down away from the ears, and keep chest open. Maintain connection of ribcage – avoid splaying.

Variations

- Progress to shoulder bridge

Exercise 4.3 Supine lying shoulder bridge (levels 2/3/4)

See Ex. 4.3

Purpose

- Spine mobility – flexion and extension
- Strengthen abdominals, gluteals, hamstrings abductors, back extensors
- Activate multifidus
- Sequential control
- Pelvic stability
- Trunk stability (when other leg movements are added at top of range)

Start position

Supine crook lying – with heels a little closer to buttocks

Note: No block.

Instructions and teaching points

1. Inhale to prepare.
2. Exhale, engage abdominals, tilt pelvis so that back flattens towards floor, engage gluteals and sequentially roll each vertebra off the floor into bridge position.

Note: At top of position, there should be a straight line from knee, through hip to armpit. The ribs should not be splayed and there should be a space between shoulders and ears.

1. Inhale at top, maintaining engagement.
2. Exhale to sequentially roll down through each vertebra and back to neutral.

Ensure chest stays open, ribcage not splaying, equal pressure through feet, shoulders down and away from ears.

Variations

- Perform pelvic tilt first and progressively build range of motion. Place a block between knees if knees roll in or out and to strengthen adductors.
- Can add heel raises and leg extensions at top of movement to challenge pelvic stability and strength of abductors (see Fig. 4.3b).

Ex. 4.3a	**Supine lying shoulder bridge**

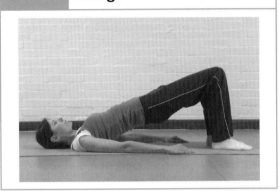

Ex. 4.3b	**Variations**

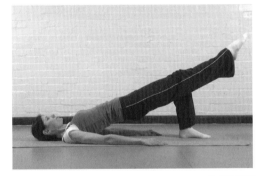

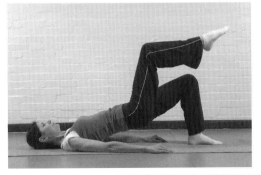

Exercise 4.4 Modified standing roll down (levels 2/3/4)

See Ex. 4.4

Purpose

- Spine mobility – flexion and extension
- Sequential control
- Pelvic stability
- Activate multifidus

Start position

Standing

Instructions and teaching points

1. Inhale to prepare and lengthen through the spine.
2. Exhale, engage abdominals and lengthen through neck, allowing chin to roll down to the chest.
3. Allow hands to hang lightly, and sequentially roll down through spine to a 45-degree angle.
4. Inhale at the bottom.
5. Exhale, engage abdominals and sequentially roll each vertebra up, stacking one on top of the other to upright position.

Variations

- Just chin tilt initially. Progressively build range of motion to 45 degrees.

Ex. 4.4	Modified standing roll down

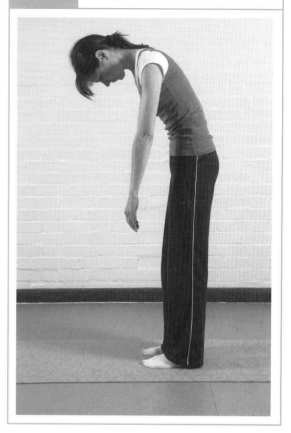

Exercise 4.5 Modified seated roll back – 'c' curve (all levels)

See Ex. 4.5

Purpose

- Spine mobility
- Pelvic and scapular stability
- Trunk stability
- Strengthen abdominals

Start position

Seated with knees bent (crook) or legs crossed

Note: Can be seated on a block for persons unable to sit on to sitting bones.

Instructions and teaching points

1. Inhale to prepare, lengthening upwards with head reaching towards ceiling.
2. Exhale, engage abdominals, keep hips as relaxed as possible. Roll the pelvis backwards, creating a rounding of the lower spine.

Note: You will feel the weight of your body travel backwards and off the sitting bones. Inhale and hold position, maintain abdominal engagement.

3. Exhale to return, visualising head being on a piece of string and lifted back up to the ceiling.

Ensure the abdominals do not dome and that the ribcage is not allowed to slump towards the pelvis.

Keep the shoulders down away from the ears and avoid letting the chin poke forwards.

Keep hip flexor muscles as relaxed as possible.

Roll back only to about 45 degrees.

Variations

- Smaller range of motion initially and progressively build range
- Can progress to performing on a stability ball

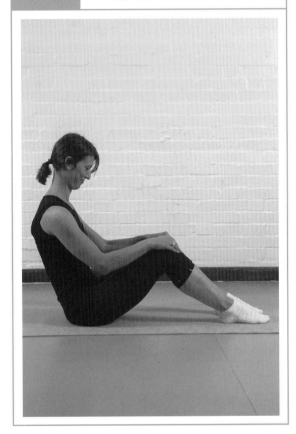

Ex. 4.5	**Modified seated roll back – 'c' curve**

Exercise 4.6 Supine hip rolls (all levels)

See Ex. 4.6

Purpose

- Pelvic stability
- Spine mobility
- Scapular stability
- Ribcage placement
- Isolation of movement
- Abdominal strength

Start position

Supine crook lying, with ankles and knees together

Instructions and teaching points

1. Inhale to prepare.
2. Exhale, engage abdominals, and rotate body lightly to one side, maintaining neutral pelvic alignment and keeping feet and knees connected together.
3. Inhale and hold at bottom.
4. Exhale, engage abdominals and return to start position.
5. Repeat other side.

Ensure ribcage does not splay. Visualise a clock face above the knees with 12 o'clock top central and 9 o'clock and 3 o'clock at the respective sides.

Variations

- Smaller range of motion to start – 5 minutes to and 5 minutes past on visualised clock face. Progress range by moving to 10 minutes to and 10 minutes past.

Ex. 4.6	Supine hip rolls

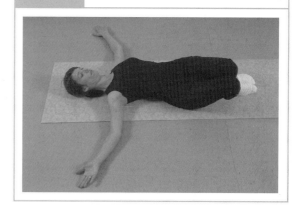

Exercise 4.7 Supine curl-up (levels 2/3/4)

See Ex. 4.7

Purpose

- Trunk stability
- Pelvic stability and maintain neutral
- Abdominal strength
- Shoulder stability to keep alignment
- Strengthen neck flexors

Start position

Supine crook lying

Instructions and teaching points

1. Inhale to prepare and tilt head to lengthen back of neck. Chin tilts gently in towards chest.
2. Exhale, engage abdominals and reach fingers towards ankles to the point where trunk lifts slightly off the floor.
3. Inhale and maintain abdominal connection.
4. Exhale to lower.

Note: Aim to maintain neutral alignment of the spine. A soft imprinting movement is okay. Watch out for excessive tilting or movement of the pelvis, use of the hip flexors and gluteals and overuse of the chest to lift the head and shoulders. Draw the scapula back and down towards the buttocks.

Variations

- Without lifting shoulders is first stage.
- Vary breathing: inhale to prepare, exhale to lift, inhale to lower.
- Vary start position to supine with legs raised (table top). Can then progress to single leg stretch.
- Progress to adapted one hundred.

Ex. 4.7	Supine curl-up

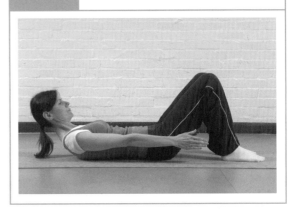

Exercise 4.8 Supine modified one hundred (levels 3/4)

See Ex. 4.8

Purpose

- Trunk stability
- Pelvic stability and maintain neutral
- Abdominal endurance
- Shoulder stability to keep alignment
- Strength and endurance of neck flexors

Start position

Supine crook lying

Instructions and teaching points

1. Inhale to prepare and tilt head to lengthen back of neck. Chin tilts in towards chest.
2. Exhale, engage abdominals and reach fingers towards ankles to the point where trunk lifts slightly off the floor. Hold position and abdominal connection.
3. Inhale 4 or 5 breaths, holding position, and wiggle fingers. Be careful not to bounce upper body and compromise shoulder alignment.
4. Exhale 4 or 5 breaths, holding position, and wiggle thumbs. Take care not to bounce upper body and compromise shoulder alignment.
5. Build to holding for count of 100.

Note: Abdominals should not round into a dome shape. Aim to maintain neutral alignment of the spine. A soft imprinting movement is okay. Watch out for excessive tilting or movement of the pelvis, use of the hip flexors and gluteals and overuse of the chest to lift the head and shoulders. Draw the scapulae back and down towards the buttocks.

Variations

- Perform with legs in table top position and light imprint if desired.

- Advance to performing in table top with neutral.
- Build repetitions progressively as position progresses. For example, when progressing to harder position, decrease repetitions initially and build these steadily.

Ex. 4.8a	Supine modified one hundred

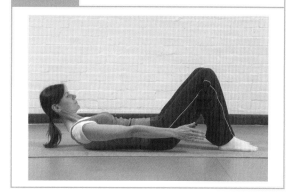

Ex. 4.8b	Variation

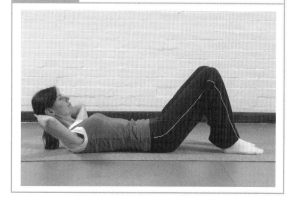

Exercise 4.9 Supine single leg stretch (levels 3/4)

See Ex. 4.9

Purpose

- Trunk stability
- Pelvic stability and maintain neutral
- Abdominal strength/endurance
- Shoulder stability to keep alignment
- Strength and endurance of neck flexors
- Strength and endurance of hip flexor muscles
- Hip mobility

Starting position

Supine lying, with knees in table top with option of light imprint or neutral

Instructions and teaching points

Advanced version

1. Inhale to prepare and tilt head to lengthen back of neck and gently move chin towards chest.
2. Exhale, engage abdominals and reach fingers forwards to the point where trunk lifts slightly off the floor.
3. Inhale and hold position, placing hands to each side of one knee.
4. Exhale, engage abdominals and extend leg, allowing the outside hand to slide down the outside of the lower leg to help keep lower leg aligned.
5. Inhale to return.
6. Exhale, engage abdominals and extend other leg.
7. Repeat.
   Keep chest open, shoulders relaxed, elbows open throughout.

Variations

- Can perform leg movements alone initially without lifting trunk:
  (1) raising leg to ceiling
  (2) extending leg slightly away from body
  (3) extending leg further away from body.
- With trunk lift, start by:
  (1) extending leg to ceiling to keep long lever over centre of gravity
  (2) extend lever slightly away from body's centre of gravity
  (3) extend leg further.

Note: The sliding arm positioning described in instructions would only need to occur for the version described above. For the variations, the hands can be held at each side of the bent knee without sliding action.

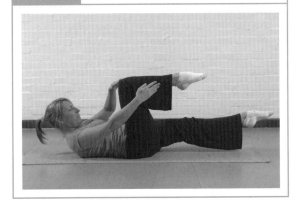

Ex. 4.9 Supine single leg stretch

Exercise 4.10 Shell/child pose stretch (all levels)

See Ex. 4.10

Purpose

- Stretch back – erector spinae and gluteals
- Stretch sides of back if arms extended in front of the body
- Stretch anterior deltoid and pectorals if shoulders pressed towards the floor
- Stretch adductors if knees taken wider
- Rest and relaxation between hands and knees exercises
- Can be used to develop lateral breathing as abdominals are restricted

Start position

Hands and knees

Instructions and teaching points

1. Inhale to prepare.
2. Exhale, engage abdominals and slide buttocks towards the heels.
3. Inhale and hold.
4. Exhale and either extend arms along the floor or allow them to slide to sides of the body – child pose.
5. Hold position and breathe laterally.
6. Return on exhale.

Variations

- Form two fists with the hands. Place one on top of the other and underneath the forehead to support the head and neck, or place a block under the head for kyphotic postures (4.10b).
- Keep the buttocks slightly away from the knees if flexibility of the spine is limited or there's any discomfort in the knees. Placing a cushion between the buttocks and the legs may help.

- Persons with knee discomfort can perform this exercise lying on one side.
- Take the legs apart slightly and lengthen the chest towards the floor to achieve a stretch of the inner thigh and pectoral muscles.

Ex. 4.10a   Shell/child pose stretch

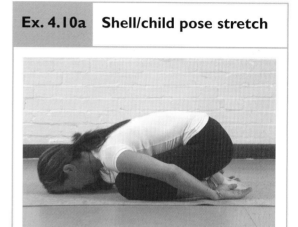

Ex. 4.10b   Variation

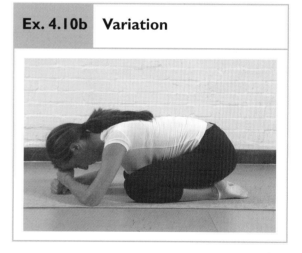

Exercise 4.11 Supine lower back release (all levels)

See Ex. 4.11

Purpose

- Lengthen erector spinae and gluteals
- Rest and relaxation between supine crook lying exercises
- Release tension and massage lower back

Start position

Supine lying, with knees held into chest

Instructions and teaching points

1. Breathe naturally.
2. Soften back into the floor – imprinting down.
3. Circle the knees lightly in one direction to release tension in the back muscles.
4. Repeat in other direction.
5. Visualise a pencil on the knees, drawing a circle on the ceiling.

Variations

- Light rocking side to side
- Light rocking forwards and backwards

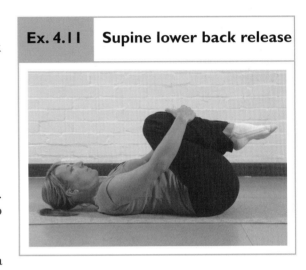

Ex. 4.11 | Supine lower back release

Exercise 4.12 Hands and knees cat stretch (all levels)

See Ex. 4.12

Purpose

- Spine mobility
- Stretch back muscles – erector spinae
- Strengthen abdominals
- Pelvic stability
- Isolation and control

Start position

Hands and knees

Instructions and teaching points

Half cat

1. Inhale to prepare.
2. Exhale, engage abdominals and tilt tail bone under, keeping upper back aligned.
3. Inhale to return to neutral or hollow back to achieve flat back posture.

Full cat

1. Inhale to prepare.
2. Exhale and engage abdominals, and round whole spine upwards – keep shoulders sliding down towards buttocks.
3. Inhale to return to neutral, or hollow back slightly for flat back posture.

Variations

- Half cat to full cat to progress mobility/range of motion

Note: From a teaching perspective, it may be easier to teach full cat first as this requires less isolation and control. Half cat demands maintenance of scapular position and upper spine alignment.

Ex. 4.12a   Half cat stretch

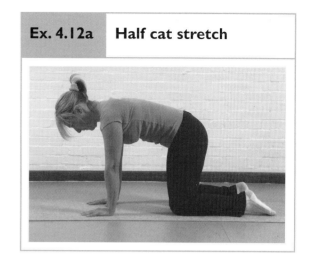

Ex. 4.12b   Full cat stretch

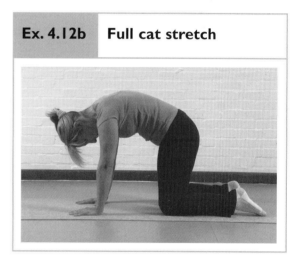

Exercise 4.13 Seated side bend (all levels)

See Ex. 4.13

Purpose

- Lengthen and stretch oblique muscles
- Pelvic stability
- Scapular stability

Start position

Seated

Instructions and teaching points

1. Inhale to prepare.
2. Exhale, engage abdominals, lengthen spine and raise arm laterally to an overhead position.
3. Inhale at the top, ensure ribcage is aligned and shoulder relaxed and down away from the ear.
4. Exhale and bend sideways to stretch the side of the body, not leaning forwards or back.
5. Hold position and breathe laterally, maintaining abdominal and scapular connections.
6. Return on an exhale.

Variations

- Lying and standing lateral arm slides to prepare for alignment of scapulae
- Perform standing up (4.13b)

Ex. 4.13a	Seated side bend

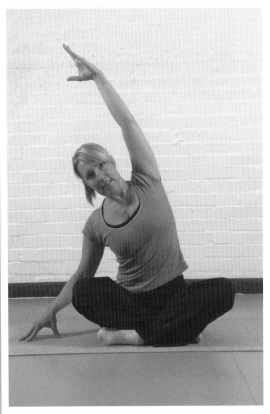

Ex. 4.13b	Standing side bend

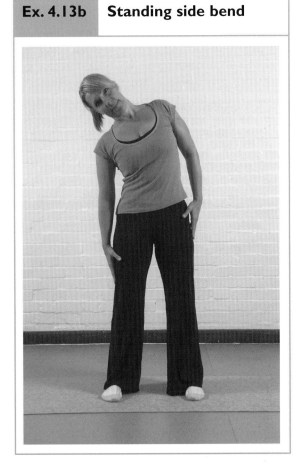

Exercise 4.14 Side plank (levels 2/3/4)

See Ex. 4.14

Purpose

- Awareness and felt connection between shoulder girdle, pelvic girdle and arm movements
- Shoulder and pelvic stability
- Trunk stability
- Strengthen muscles between shoulder blades
- Ribcage placement
- Upper body strength (support arm)
- Lengthen oblique muscles when arm outstretched

Start position

Side half-lying, with crook knees (bent) and heels aligned with buttocks. Lower arm should be bent and elbow positioned under shoulder, with hand in front of body and top arm lengthening down over top hip.

Instructions and teaching points

1. Inhale to prepare, pelvis neutral, shoulders lengthening down away from ears and shoulder blades sliding towards buttocks.
2. Exhale, engage abdominals, strengthen connection at shoulder blades (not dropping forwards) and between ribs and hips.
3. Raise lower buttock off the floor.
4. At the same time, raise the top arm in a lateral action over the head (keeping a space between shoulder and ear).
5. Inhale to lower, maintaining abdominal engagement.
6. Repeat both sides.

Variations

Prepare for lateral arm movement with lying and standing lateral arm slides (*see* Chapter 6 Exercises 5 and 6).

- Lengthen obliques with seated side stretch (see exercise 4.13, p. 68).
- Perform without arm reach initially
- Perform with legs extended straight out to the side of the body with all joints aligned (see Fig. 4.14b)

Ex. 4.14a	Side plank

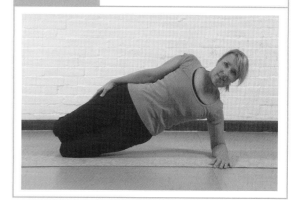

Ex. 4.14b	Advanced side plank

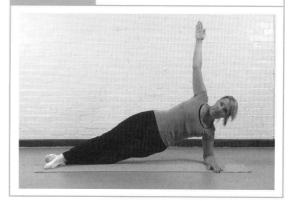

THE PELVIC GIRDLE AND PELVIC FLOOR

5

Structure of the pelvic girdle

The pelvic girdle is part of the appendicular skeleton. It is formed from the joining of two innominate (sometimes called coxal, pelvic or hip) bones (one to the right and one to the left) with the sacrum in the middle. The innominate bones on each side are themselves made from three separate bones, the ilium, ischium and pubic bones that fuse (join) together by adulthood.

The *ilium* is a broad, plate-like, curved irregular bone that forms the upper (superior) part of the innominate bone. It has a prominent upper rim called the iliac crest, which runs between the anterior superior iliac spine (ASIS) at the front of the pelvis and the posterior superior iliac spine (PSIS) at the back of the pelvis.

The iliac crest can be felt quite easily in most people (it is about 10cm above the hip joint and just below the waist area). It can also be observed in leaner, bony individuals. The ASIS is more prominent and can be felt at the front, especially in females (due to their wider pelvis). The PSIS can be felt at the back. Both the ASIS and PSIS are used to assess posture (see chapter 7).

The ASIS can also be used with the pubic bone as a landmark for individuals to find a neutral pelvic position. For example, place the heel of the hand on the ASIS and point the fingers towards the pubic bone, forming a triangle. The bones should be aligned vertically when standing and horizontally when lying.

The *ischium* or sitting bones are lower (inferior) to the ilium. They are thick and strong in order to support the body weight when sitting. The ischial tuberosities can be felt underneath the buttocks in a seated position.

The innominate bones join at the front, back and sides to form the pelvic bowl:

At the back (posterior), they join with the sacrum to form the load-bearing sacroiliac joint.

At the side (lateral), they form the deep cup-shaped socket (the acetabulum) into which the head of the thigh bone (the femur) fits to form the hip joint. The socket is deep and offers support and stability.

At the front (anterior), the pubic bones join together to form the cartilaginous joint, the pubis symphysis.

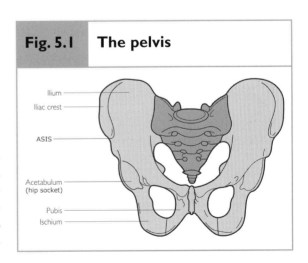

Fig. 5.1 **The pelvis**

Ilium
Iliac crest
ASIS
Acetabulum (hip socket)
Pubis
Ischium

Note: The male pelvis is narrower, with the acetebulum more vertical to assist running. The female pelvis is wider and deeper to facilitate childbirth. The acetebulum tilts back, making running actions more problematic as there is a tendency for the legs to swing out and the knees to roll inwards. This rolling inwards of the knees can sometimes be observed during squatting.

The sacroiliac joints

These occur where the iliac bones meet the sacrum at the rear of the body – right and left sides. They are considered to be both synovial (freely movable), because the lower sections have some movement, and also fibrous (immovable), because the upper sections have no movement.

Hately Aldous (2005) describes the following movements at the sacroiliac joints:

- Nutation – where the sacrum moves across the innominate bones at S2 and forwards into the pelvic bowl;
- Counternutation – where the sacrum moves across the innominate bones at S2 and backwards from the pelvic bowl.

Function of the pelvic girdle

The pelvic girdle has a number of functions:

- It supports the internal organs of the pelvic region.

- It supports the weight of the body that is transmitted through the legs (standing) and ischium (sitting).
- It provides attachment for muscles.
- It assists with correct walking action.
- It plays an important role in ensuring the correct alignment of the spine (the neutral spine position).
- It provides bony support for the birth canal in females.

Muscles supporting and moving the pelvic girdle and hip joint

A number of muscle groups attach to the pelvic girdle and mobilise the hip joint. They are:

- Quadriceps and hip flexors (anteriorly)
- Gluteus maximus and hamstrings (posteriorly)
- Abductors, tensor fascia latae, piriformis (laterally)
- Adductors, pectineus (medially)

Muscles attaching at the front of the pelvis to the thigh

Note: Refer to the major muscles diagrams on pp. 40–41 for the position of the different muscles.

Table 5.1	Hip flexor – iliopsoas
• Iliacus • Psoas minor • Psoas major	
Description and muscle action	Group of three muscles (iliacus and psoas major). Runs from both right and left sides of the body, from the iliac crest (iliacus) and vertebrae L1 to L5 and T12 (psoas major) to the top of the femur, crossing over the hip joint.
Actions:	• Hip flexion • Flexion of spine because of insertion point for psoas major (when sitting up from a lying position – Thompson 1989) • External rotation of femur (Thompson 1989) *Note:* Overactivity of this muscle without sufficient strength of the core muscles can contribute to hyperextension of the spine.

Table 5.2	Quadriceps
• Rectus femoris • Vastus medialis • Vastus intermedius • Vastus lateralis	
Description and muscle action	Large group of four muscles spanning the front and sides of the thigh, crossing the hip (rectus femoris) and knee joint (all four muscles) via the patella tendon.
Actions:	Rectus femoris • Flexes the hip (assists hip flexor/iliopsoas muscles) Vastus medialis • A key role in stabilising the knee. Works in last 15 degrees of knee extension All muscles in group • Extend the knee – with the vasti muscles primarily acting as assistants to rectus femoris

Muscles attaching from the back of the pelvis to the thigh

Note: Refer to the major muscles diagrams on pp. 40–41 for the position of the different muscles.

Table 5.3	Gluteus maximus (hip extensors)
Description and muscle action	Large, thick band of muscle on both sides of the body (posterior), forming the buttocks. Runs from the base of the spine and pelvis (sacrum, coccyx and ilium) to the top and back (posterior) of the thigh bone (femur).
Actions:	• Extension of the hip – 'comes into action when movement between the pelvis and femur approaches and goes beyond 15 degrees' (Thompson, 1989:68) • Lateral (outward) rotation of the hip.

Table 5.4	Hamstrings
• Biceps femoris • Semitendinosus • Semimembranosus	
Description and muscle action	Group of three muscles crossing over the hip and knee at the rear of the thigh.
Actions:	• Extension of the hip • Inward (medial) rotation of hip (semitendinosus and semimembranosus) • Outward (lateral) rotation of hip (biceps femoris) • Flexion of the knee (Thompson, 1989 and Stone & Stone, 1990)

Muscles attaching from the outside of the pelvis to the pelvis

Note: Refer to the major muscles diagrams on pp. 40–41 for the position of the different muscles.

Table 5.5	Abductors
• Gluteus medius (medium size) • Gluteus minimus (small size)	
Description and muscle action	Deeper than gluteus maximus, extending from the side of the ilium to the top side of the femur, crossing the hip joint.
Actions:	• Abducts the hip • Inward (medial) rotation as hip abducts (gluteus minimus and anterior fibres of the medius muscle) • Outward rotation as the hip abducts (posterior fibres of gluteus medius)

Table 5.6	Piriformis
Description and muscle action	Running through each side of the pelvis from the sacrum to the outer top ridge of the femur (greater trochanter).
Actions:	• Outward (lateral) rotation of thigh/hip • Abduction of hip (Stone and Stone, 1990)

Table 5.7	Tensor fascia latae
Description and muscle action	Small, thick muscle embedded in the top of the anterior lateral fascia. Runs from side of the iliac crest to the iliotibial band of the outer thigh, which then inserts into the tibia condyle.
Actions:	• Flexion of hip • Inward (medial) rotation of hip as it flexes • Horizontal abduction of hip • Stabilises the pelvis by pulling on fascia that runs down the side of the thigh (Thompson, 1989:65)

Muscles attaching from the pelvis to the inner thigh

Note: Refer to the major muscles diagrams on pp. 40–41 for the position of the different muscles.

Table 5.8	Adductors
• Adductor longus (long) • Adductor magnus (thick) • Adductor brevis (short/brief)	
Description and muscle action	Triangular band of three muscles, spanning from the pubis to the inside of the femur and crossing the hip joint.
Actions:	• Adduction of the thigh • Outward (lateral) rotation as hip adducts (adductor longus and adductor brevis) • Adductor longus assists with hip flexion

Table 5.9	Pectineus
Description and muscle action	Short band of muscle running from pubic bone to top of inner thigh bone. Sometimes grouped as a hip flexor but usually grouped as an adductor.
Actions:	• Flexion of hip • Adduction of hip • Internal rotation of the hip • Has no major role in stabilizing the pelvis

Table 5.9	Gracilis
Description and muscle action	Long thin strip of muscle running both sides from pubis to tibia and crossing the hip and knee. Most superficial of the hip adductors.
Actions:	• Adduction of hip • Internal rotation of the hip • Knee flexion

Theory into practice – application

When we bend forwards, sit down and stand up, all the large mobiliser muscles (hip flexors, gluteals and so on) will be involved in some way, either contracting (as the prime mover, or main muscle working) or relaxing (as the antagonist, the opposite muscle that relaxes when the prime mover contracts). To enable these movements, the sacrum moves into nutation (slightly tilts forwards into the pelvic bowl) to stabilise and accommodate the transfer of weight between the spine and the lower body (Hately Aldous, 2005).

Numerous strong ligaments support the connection of the iliac bones with the sacrum to prevent unnecessary movement. These ligaments, in conjunction with the muscles that attach to the pelvis (from both the upper and lower body), help maintain the integrity of the pelvis (keep it together and stable).

Excessive weakness or tightness of the ligaments and/or muscular structures around the pelvis and sacroiliac joints can have an impact on this integrity. For example, during pregnancy the ligaments may become more mobile to enable child birth, thereby reducing stability in this area.

Mobility problems at the hip joint (due to excessive tightness or weakness of any of the surrounding muscles – hip flexors, abductors, hamstrings and deeper muscles), or problems within the spine (poor core stability), may contribute to tightening of the ligaments supporting the pelvis and lead to further restriction of movement and mobility.

Weak core muscles and poor posture (lordosis, flat back) will also have an effect on the alignment of the spine in relation to the pelvis and contribute to dysfunctional movement patterns. For more information, see chapter 7 on posture and posture types.

The sciatic and gluteal nerves, and a number of other nerves, leave the spinal column in the pelvic region to connect with the lower body. Thus any related problem (tightness or weakness) can result in these nerves becoming compressed.

Balance between the strength and flexibility of the mobiliser muscles surrounding the pelvis is essential to promote functional movement and correct alignment and posture.

The main muscles that contribute to stability of the sacroiliac joints are the stabiliser muscles: transverses abdominis, multifidus and the pelvic floor. Thus synchronicity between the working of these muscles is essential. As explained at the end of chapter 4, Pilates encourages engagement of these core muscles.

The pelvic floor muscles

The pelvic floor consists of a number of muscles (including levator ani and coccygeus) that run underneath the pelvis like a hammock on both right and left sides to surround the lower orifices: the urethra and vagina (females) and penis and testes (male), and the anus.

The fibres of the pelvic floor muscles run backwards, downwards and inwards from the back (coccyx and ischial spine) to the front (pubic bone). They connect centrally, inserting into the perineal body, the sides of the anal canal and the ligament between the anus and the coccyx. They are separated centrally by the male prostate and the female vagina (Palastanga et al, 1990).

Fig. 5.2 The pelvic floor muscles

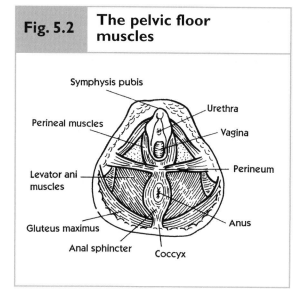

These muscles form the lower part of the inner cylinder and will impact the effectiveness of the abdominal balloon mechanism described in chapter 4. They have a number of important functions, which include:

- Supporting the contents of the pelvis and abdomen
- Contracting to maintain continence when intra-abdominal pressure changes (for example, when coughing, sneezing, laughing)
- Helping to increase intra-abdominal pressure
- Maintaining bladder control and helping to expel urine
- Preventing stress incontinence
- Maintaining bowel continence and expelling faeces
- Helping to expel semen
- Preventing prolapse (sagging of the walls of the vagina) and assisting with recovery from prolapse
- Increasing enjoyment and excitement during penetrative sex and enhancing orgasm

A number of factors can cause the pelvic floor to become weakened. Weakness is generally more common in females then males (Palastanga et al, 1990). These factors include:

- Pregnancy – the weight of the baby pressing against the pelvic floor
- Childbirth – stretching and tearing of the muscles
- Prolonged inactivity
- Urinary diseases and infections
- Constipation and other bowel conditions (irritable bowel)
- Obesity
- Excessive coughing (some respiratory conditions)
- Excessive and sustained jumping and impact
- Hormonal changes (pregnancy and menopause)
- Prostatectomy (males)
- Constant heavy lifting as required by some occupations, causing continual pressure on these muscles

Tests for sensitivity and control of the pelvic floor

During penetrative sex, the female can squeeze the pelvic floor muscles against her partner's penis (Dale and Roeber, 1984).

During urination, try stopping the flow. The muscles are okay if you can stop and restart the flow. Empty your bladder fully after this exercise (Dale and Roeber, 1984).

Males can squeeze the band of muscle around the penis and the back of the scrotum like squeezing a ball, to 'lift' the penis.

Pelvic floor exercises

These can be performed in a relaxed supine crook lying position, prone lying position or in a seated position. They can also be performed while standing and practised during daily activities (for example, while standing in a queue or walking). Care should be taken not to squeeze the muscles around the thighs or buttocks.

A large percentage (approximately 70 per cent) of the pelvic floor muscles are slow twitch fibres (slow to contract and slow to tire, and designed for endurance). A smaller percentage (approximately 30 per cent) are fast twitch (fast to contract and fast to tire, and designed for strength). It is therefore suggested that you include a combination of slower exercises for the pelvic floor (like the lift/elevator) and faster exercises (light switch and passage isolations) to recruit both types of fibre.

Robinson (2000:33) recommends recruiting these muscles at 30 per cent of maximum contraction. She also suggests, as a way of engaging the muscle, 'to suck the thumb as you draw them up inside'.

Back passage squeeze

Inhale to prepare and exhale to isolate and draw up the muscles of the pelvic floor surrounding the anus – without gripping the buttocks or other muscles. Inhale to release.

Middle passage squeeze

Inhale to prepare and exhale to isolate and draw up the muscles of the pelvic floor surrounding the vagina – without gripping the buttocks or other muscles. Inhale to release.

Front passage squeeze

Inhale to prepare and exhale to isolate and draw up the muscles of the pelvic floor surrounding the urethra – without gripping the buttocks or other muscles. Inhale to release.

Back to front – the wave

Inhale to prepare and exhale to draw up the muscles of the pelvic floor surrounding the anus, vagina and urethra sequentially – without gripping the buttocks. Inhale to release.

Front to back – the reverse wave

Inhale to prepare and exhale to draw up the muscles of the pelvic floor surrounding the urethra, vagina and anus sequentially – without gripping the buttocks. Inhale to release.

The flower – for isolation of each orifice

Visualise each orifice of the pelvic floor as an 'open flower'. Inhale to prepare and exhale to draw the muscles around the orifice upwards to close the petals of the flower.

The flower

Visualise the whole of the pelvic floor area between the legs as an 'open flower'. Inhale to prepare and exhale to draw the muscles upwards to close the petals of the flower, feeling also the connection with the deeper abdominals.

The light switch

Inhale to prepare. Exhale to draw up the pelvic floor muscles (either just one, or all sequentially, or all together), visualising the light switching on. Inhale to release, visualising the light switching off.

The lift or elevator

Females:
- Visualise the vagina as a lift shaft with three floors – ground, middle and top.

- Inhale to prepare and visualise the doors of the lift opening on the ground floor and a person entering the lift.
- Exhale and engage the pelvic floor. Draw the muscles up, visualising the lift closing and then rising to the second floor.
- Inhale, holding the contraction steady, and visualise the doors of the lift opening again on the middle floor and more people entering.
- Exhale and draw the pelvic floor upwards again, visualising the doors closing and the lift travelling to the top floor.
- Inhale and hold the contraction, visualising the lift doors opening and some people getting out and others getting in.
- Exhale to lower the lift down to the middle floor again (this is the hardest to control).
- Inhale as the door opens at the middle floor and people transfer in and out.
- Exhale, allowing the lift to travel to the ground floor.
- Relax.

Males:
- Inhale to prepare
- Exhale and tighten the band of muscle around the penis and the scrotum (like squeezing or gripping a ball). The penis may lift
- Inhale and hold the contraction
- Exhale and draw the muscles up further
- Inhale and hold the contraction
- Exhale and release the squeezing action slightly
- Inhale and hold the contraction
- Exhale and release the squeezing action
- Relax

(These details are taken from Robinson, 2000 and Latey, 2001.)

Modified exercises

Exercise 5.1 Supine crook lying heel slide (all levels)

See Ex. 5.1

Purpose

- Develop awareness and felt connection between pelvic girdle and hip
- Pelvic stability
- Hip mobility
- Trunk stability
- Ribcage placement
- Movement isolation

Start position

Supine crook lying

The legs need to be able to slide along the floor, so perform the exercise with socks on. This will allow the foot to slide along the floor.

Instructions and teaching points

1. Inhale to prepare.
2. Exhale, engage abdominals and, without moving the pelvis, slide the leg along the floor. If you feel the pelvis wanting to move, avoid going any further. Inhale at the bottom.
3. Exhale, engage abdominals and slide the leg back to its original position.

Make sure the legs do not lift off the floor.

Variations

- Place the hands on the pelvic bones (to monitor movement of the pelvis)
- One leg at a time
- Alternate legs
- Combine with overhead arm floats – see p. 110

Ex. 5.1	Supine crook lying heel slide

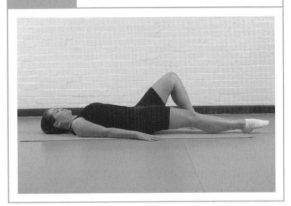

Exercise 5.2 Supine heel raise (all levels)

See Ex. 5.2

Purpose

- Trunk stability
- Pelvic stability
- Isolation of movement
- Ankle mobility
- Slight hip mobility

Start position

Supine crook lying

Instructions and teaching points

1. Inhale to prepare.
2. Exhale, engage abdominals, maintain pelvic alignment and raise one heel from the floor, keeping the ball of the foot on the floor.
3. Inhale to return.

Variations

- One leg at a time
- Alternate legs
- Both heels together
- Progress to knee raise

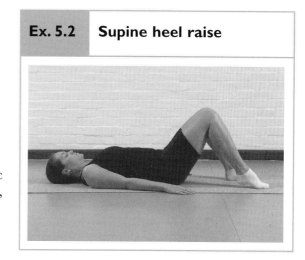

Ex. 5.2	Supine heel raise

Exercise 5.3 Supine knee raise/float (all levels)

See Ex. 5.3

Purpose

- Trunk stability
- Pelvic stability
- Ribcage alignment
- Isolation of movement
- Hip mobility

Start position

Supine crook lying

Instructions and teaching points

1. Inhale to prepare.
2. Exhale, engage abdominals, maintain pelvic alignment and raise one heel from the floor to the ball of the foot and then lift the foot in an arc-like motion, so that the knee is over the hip. Keep the knee position constant.
3. Inhale and maintain abdominal engagement to return.

Variations

- Could start with feet on blocks or otherwise elevated to make it easier
- One leg at a time
- Alternate legs
- Progress to knee drops
- Combine with arm floats – see chapter 6

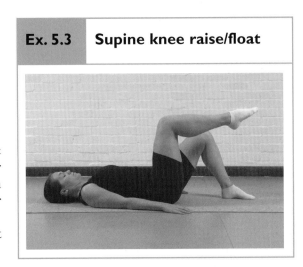

Ex. 5.3	Supine knee raise/float

Exercise 5.4 Supine toe dips from table top (levels 2/3/4)

See Ex. 5.4

Purpose

- Trunk stability
- Pelvic stability
- Ribcage alignment
- Isolation of movement
- Hip mobility

Start position

Supine lying, with knees elevated and aligned over hips (table top). Keep the knees bent at a 90-degree angle.

Spine can be either neutral or with light imprint.

Instructions and teaching points

1. Inhale to prepare.
2. Exhale, engage abdominals and connect with ribcage (not allowing ribs to lift).
3. Lower one foot towards the floor as if dipping toe into a bowl of water.
4. Inhale to lift and return.

Variations

- One leg at a time
- Alternate legs
- Progress by taking leg further away, lengthening lever
- Combine with overhead arm floats – see chapter 6

Ex. 5.4	Supine toe dips from table top

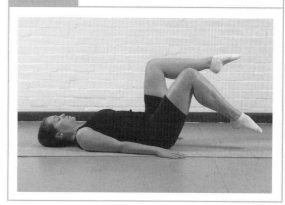

Exercise 5.5 Hands and knees leg raise/extension (levels 2/3/4)

See Ex. 5.5

Purpose

- Develop awareness and felt connection between pelvic girdle and hip
- Pelvic and shoulder stability
- Strengthen gluteal muscles
- Trunk stability
- Ribcage placement
- Movement isolation
- Develop balance

Start position

Hands and knees

Instructions and teaching points

1. Inhale to prepare.
2. Lengthen shoulders down away from ears, with shoulder blades sliding towards buttocks.
3. Exhale, engage abdominals, strengthen connection of pelvic girdle. Slide the leg backwards to straighten the knee so that the foot is extending back away from the body.
4. Inhale to lower.

Variations

- Can be progressed by extending the leg backwards and lifting the leg upwards towards the ceiling. Ensure pelvis remains stable and ribcage placement and shoulder girdle alignment are not compromised (see Fig. 5.5b).
- Can be progressed further by combining with arm raise – see the exercises in chapter 6.

| Ex. 5.5a | **Hands and knees leg raise/extension** |

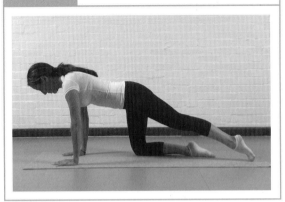

| Ex. 5.5b | **Advanced hands and knees leg raise/extension** |

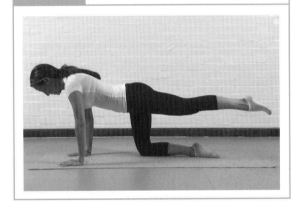

Exercise 5.6 Side lying outer thigh raise (all levels)

See Ex. 5.6

Purpose

- Develop awareness and felt connection between pelvic girdle and hip
- Pelvic stability
- Strengthen abductor muscles
- Trunk stability
- Ribcage placement
- Movement isolation
- Develop balance

Start position

Side lying

Instructions and teaching points

1. Inhale to prepare.
2. Exhale, engage abdominals, keep the waist lifted away from the floor.
3. Maintain placement of ribcage and point the foot, extending and raising the leg towards the ceiling.
4. Inhale, flex the foot, lengthen and lower the leg to start position.

Ex. 5.6a	Side lying outer thigh raise

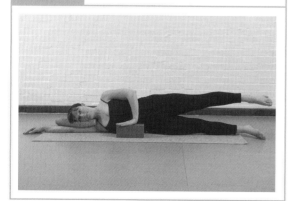

Variations

- As a starter, just pointing and flexing the foot without lifting the leg

Ex. 5.6b	Variation

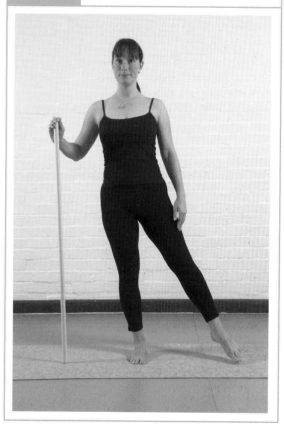

Exercise 5.7 Side lying inner thigh raise (all levels)

See Ex. 5.7

Purpose

- Develop awareness and felt connection between pelvic girdle and hip
- Pelvic stability
- Strengthen adductor muscles
- Trunk stability
- Ribcage placement
- Movement isolation

Start position

Side lying

Place top leg across the body and towards the floor, with the knee and ankle supported on either a towel or block.

Instructions and teaching points

1. Inhale to prepare.
2. Exhale, engage abdominals, keep the waist lifted away from the floor.
3. Maintain placement of ribcage and point the foot, extending and raising the lower leg towards the ceiling.
4. Inhale, flex the foot, lengthen and lower the leg to start position.

Variations

- As a starter, just pointing and flexing the foot without lifting the lower leg

Ex. 5.7b	Variation

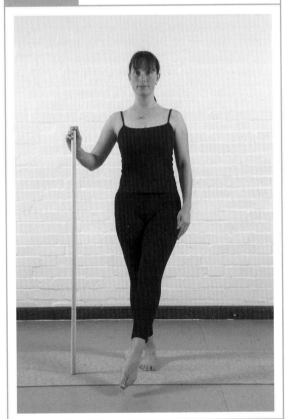

Ex. 5.7a	Side lying inner thigh raise

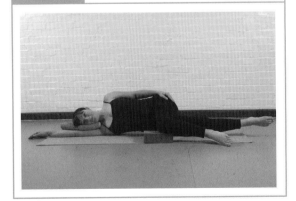

Exercise 5.8 Prone lying leg raise (all levels)

See Ex. 5.8

Purpose

- Develop awareness and felt connection between pelvic girdle and hip
- Pelvic stability
- Strengthen gluteal muscles
- Trunk stability
- Ribcage placement
- Movement isolation

Start position

Prone lying, with hands resting under forehead

Note: Towel or small arc/barrel apparatus can be used underneath abdominals as a support for persons with lordosis to reduce pull on lumbar spine.

Instructions and teaching points

1. Inhale to prepare.
2. Exhale, engage abdominals, keep the tummy button lifted upwards.
3. Maintain placement of ribcage, extending and raising the leg back and upwards.
4. Inhale, lengthen and lower the leg to start position.
5. Maintain neutral alignment and take care not to press the weight on to the opposite leg.

Variations

- One leg at a time
- Alternate legs
- Both legs together with care!

Ex. 5.8 **Prone lying leg raise**

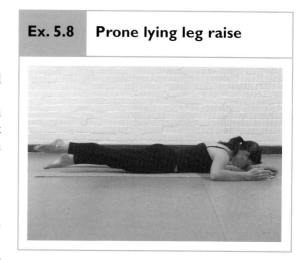

Exercise 5.9 Prone gluteal bracing (all levels)

See Ex. 5.9

Purpose

- Develop awareness and felt connection between pelvic girdle and hip
- Pelvic stability
- Strengthen gluteal muscles
- Trunk stability
- Ribcage placement
- Movement isolation
- Develop balance

Start position

Prone lying, with hands resting under forehead

Feet at hip's width, with ankles rolling out slightly

Instructions and teaching points

1. Inhale to prepare.
2. Exhale and sequentially engage abdominals – lifting tummy button upwards, tightening buttock muscles.
3. Keeping pelvis neutral, bring inner thighs and knees together.
4. With a light squeeze, draw ankles together, maintaining strong extension and lengthening of the legs.
5. Inhale at the top, maintaining abdominal connection.
6. Exhale and sequentially release ankles, knees, thighs, buttocks and, last of all, abdominals.

Variations

- Variation to the breathing – inhale to prepare, exhale to lift, inhale to lower
- Hold isometrically at the top, maintaining lateral breathing.

Ex. 5.9	Prone gluteal bracing

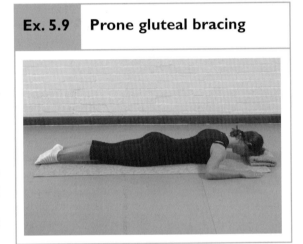

Exercise 5.10 Side lying clam (levels 2/3/4)

See Ex. 5.10

Purpose

- Develop awareness and felt connection between pelvic girdle and hip
- Pelvic and shoulder stability
- Strengthen abductor muscles
- Trunk stability
- Ribcage placement
- Movement isolation
- Develop balance

Start position

Side lying with knees crooked (bent)

Bend at hip so that knees are forward of the body with heels aligned with the coccyx

Upper ankles, knees and hip should be stacked directly above lower ankles, knees and hip

Instructions and teaching points

1. Inhale to prepare.
2. Exhale, engage abdominals, keep the waist lifted away from the floor.
3. Maintain placement of ribcage (taking care not to protrude forwards), and keeping ankles touching, lightly raise and rotate the top knee outwards and backwards.
4. Inhale and hold at the top and maintain abdominal engagement.
5. Exhale and lower the leg to start position.

Variations

- Variation to the breathing – inhale to prepare, exhale to lift, inhale to lower.

Ex. 5.10	Side lying clam

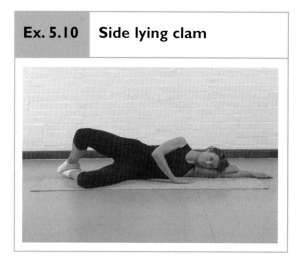

Exercise 5.11 Supine ankle bends and foot circles (all levels)

See Ex. 5.11

Purpose

- Pelvic stability
- Trunk stability and ribcage placement
- Ankle mobility
- Strengthen hip flexor and quadriceps
- Actively lengthen hamstring in extended position

Start position

Supine crook lying

Instructions and teaching points

1. Inhale to prepare.
2. Exhale and engage abdominals.
3. Float one leg upwards so that knee is over hip, and keep lower leg parallel to ceiling.
4. Inhale and hold position.
5. Exhale and point toe.
6. Inhale to flex foot.
7. Repeat.
8. Return on an exhale.
9. Repeat on other leg.

Variations

- Progress to holding knee joint straight so that the toe points to the ceiling
- Perform foot circles in both positions
- Perform small leg circles in both positions
  a) With bent leg, visualise having a pencil on knee and drawing a circle on ceiling
  b) With leg straight, visualise having pencil between toes

Note: Keep circle small and evenly shaped – maximum 12 inches circumference.

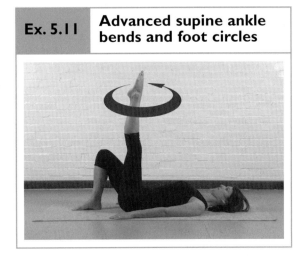

| Ex. 5.11 | **Advanced supine ankle bends and foot circles** |

Exercise 5.12 Lying hamstring stretch (all levels)

See Ex. 5.12

Purpose

- Stretch the hamstrings
- Develop awareness and felt connection between pelvic girdle and hip joint
- Pelvic and trunk stability to hold alignment

Start position

Supine crook lying

Instructions and teaching points

1. Inhale to prepare.
2. Exhale, engage abdominals and keep the pelvis in a neutral position.
3. Raise the leg to a point where a mild tension is felt at the back of the thigh. Aim to extend the knee fully on the stretching leg and hold the back of the thigh.
4. Hold the position and breathe laterally.
5. Keep the head and shoulders supported on the floor.
6. Keep the knee joint of the other leg bent.
7. Return on an exhale.

Variations

- Place a strap around the foot to assist the stretch.
- When holding the stretch, the stretch can be increased further on the exhale by drawing the leg straighter or closer towards the body (care should be taken to maintain the neutral alignment and to avoid the back sinking to the floor as this may promote greater stretch of the gluteals and back muscles and decrease the stretch of the hamstrings).
- Develop the stretch by holding for an increased duration when in extended position.

Ex. 5.12a Lying hamstring stretch

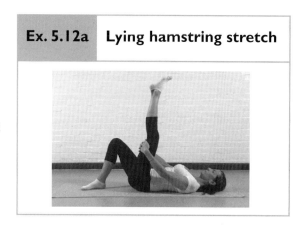

Ex. 5.12b Lying hamstring stretch with strap

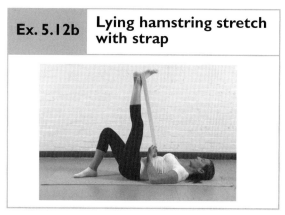

Ex. 5.12c Standing hamstring stretch

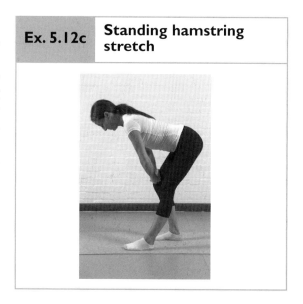

Exercise 5.13 Lying quadriceps stretch (all levels)

See Ex. 5.13

Purpose

- Stretch the quadriceps
- Develop awareness and felt connection between pelvic girdle and hip joint
- Pelvic and trunk stability to hold alignment

Start position

Prone lying or side lying

Instructions and teaching points

1. Inhale to prepare.
2. Exhale, engage abdominals and lift the lower leg towards the buttocks to a point where a mild tension is felt at the front of the thigh. Do not over flex (bend) the knee. The ankle can be held by the hand.
3. Lift the heel towards the centre of the buttock cheeks, avoid taking the heel to the outside of the buttocks as this may stress the ligaments on the inside of the knee.
4. Hold position and breathe laterally.
5. Keep the hips facing forwards and avoid hollowing of the lower back.
6. Return on an exhale.

Variations

- Use a strap around the ankle to assist the stretch
- Side lying may be easier for persons lacking flexibility
- Stretching both legs together when prone is a method for progressing the stretch

Ex. 5.13a   Lying quadriceps stretch

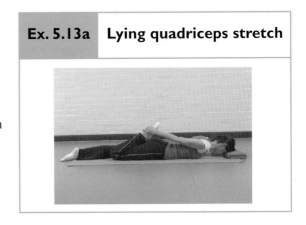

Ex. 5.13b   Side lying quadriceps stretch

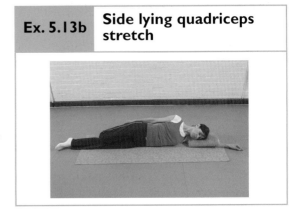

Ex. 5.13c   Standing quadriceps stretch

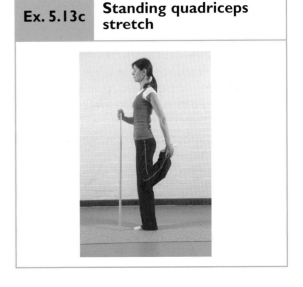

Exercise 5.14 Seated adductor stretch (all levels)

See Ex. 5.14

Purpose

- Stretch the adductors
- Develop awareness and felt connection between pelvic girdle and ribcage
- Trunk stability to hold alignment

Start position

Seated on floor

Instructions and teaching points

1. Inhale to prepare.
2. Exhale, engage abdominals and slide the legs to the side of the body to a straddle position (hands can be on the floor supporting the body weight).
3. Hold position and breathe laterally.

Ensure you're sitting on the sitting bones and lifting out of the pelvis, lengthening the spine. Keep a space between the ribs and hips and don't allow the centre to collapse.

4. Return on an exhale.

Variations

- Perform with soles of feet together and dropping knees out to each side again. The hands can be placed behind the body to help maintain an upright seated position. The stretch can be increased this way by pressing the weight forwards with the hands to increase upright sitting and encourage legs to move further down.
- Sit on a block if flexibility does not allow an upright sitting position to be maintained (for example, those with flat back posture).
- Start with a smaller range of motion and progress the range by taking the legs further in the straddle position.

- Soles of feet together can be progressed by holding ankles (or keeping hands on floor), bringing the feet closer towards the pubic bone.

Ex. 5.14a   Seated adductor stretch

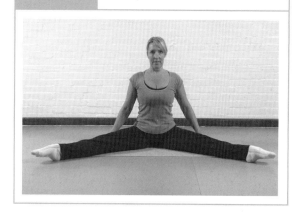

Ex. 5.14b   Alternative seated adductor stretch

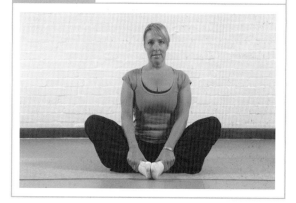

Exercise 5.15 Seated hamstring stretch (all levels)

See Ex. 5.15

Purpose

- Stretch the hamstrings
- Develop awareness and felt connection between pelvic girdle and rib cage
- Trunk stability to hold alignment

Start position

Seated, with one leg straight out in front of the body and the other knee bent in a comfortable position

Instructions and teaching points

1. Inhale to prepare and sit upright on the sitting bones, with one leg extended in front of the body and the other in a comfortable position at the side of the body.
2. Keep the knee of the leg to be stretched straight but not locked. The hands can be placed at the side of the extended leg as support.
3. Exhale, engage abdominals and lengthen the spine.
4. Visualise lifting the body upwards and forwards out of the hips (bending from the hip not the spine).
5. The hands can slide steadily forwards, maintaining connection of shoulder girdle (not slouching or hunching).

6. Stretch to a point where a mild tension is felt at the back of the thigh.
7. Hold position and maintain lateral breathing.
8. Take care not to tense front of thigh.
9. Return upright on an exhale.

Variations

- Start by only bending a little way forwards.
- Progress by bending over slightly further to achieve a greater range of motion.
- Push the buttocks backwards further on the stretching leg to increase the stretch.

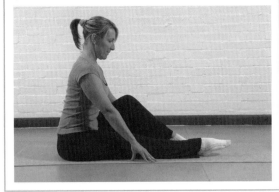

Ex. 5.15   **Seated hamstring stretch**

Exercise 5.16 Kneeling hip flexor stretch (levels 2/3/4)

See Ex. 5.16

Purpose

- Stretch the hip flexor
- Develop awareness and felt connection between pelvic girdle and ribcage
- Trunk stability to hold alignment
- Maintain balance

Start position

Kneeling

Instructions and teaching points

1. Inhale to prepare.
2. Exhale, engage abdominals and lunge one foot out to the front with the foot on the floor.
3. Inhale at the top.
4. Exhale, engage abdominals, lengthen the spine upwards, keeping pelvis neutral and hips squared to front.
5. Take the body weight slightly forwards into the stretch.
6. Keep the knee of the front leg in line over the ankle and ensure the knee does not overshoot the toe.
7. Hold the position and breathe laterally.
8. Exhale and engage abdominals to return leg inwards.

Variations

- Place a towel under support knee for more comfort.
- Less flexible participants can perform this stretch standing up, with one leg back slightly and the hips tilted forwards. This can be progressed gradually by progressively taking the leg further back and sinking the body weight down towards the floor.

| Ex. 5.16a | **Kneeling hip flexor stretch** |

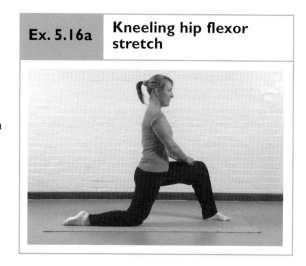

| Ex. 5.16b | **Standing hip flexor stretch** |

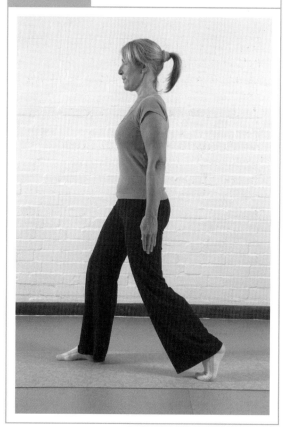

Exercise 5.17 Supine lying hip flexor stretch (all levels)

See Ex. 5.17

Purpose

- Stretch the hip flexor
- Develop awareness and felt connection between pelvic girdle and ribcage
- Pelvic alignment
- Trunk stability to hold alignment
- Maintain balance

Start position

Supine crook lying

Instructions and teaching points

1. Inhale to prepare.
2. Exhale, engage abdominals and raise one knee towards the chest, taking hold of the back of the thigh.
3. Maintain pelvic alignment (not rising on one side), and keep equal space between ribs and hips.
4. Inhale and hold at the top.
5. Exhale, engage abdominals and slide leg on floor to a fully extended position. Visualise someone pulling leg away from body.
6. Hold position and breathe laterally.
7. On exhalation, return lower leg to bent position and top leg to floor.

Variations

- Place a towel or block under extended knee for persons with less flexibility

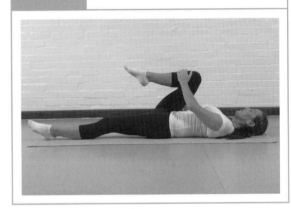

Ex. 5.17   **Supine lying hip flexor stretch**

Exercise 5.18 Seated abductor stretch (all levels)

See Ex. 5.18

Purpose

- Stretch the abductors
- Develop awareness and felt connection between pelvic girdle and ribcage
- Pelvic alignment
- Pelvic stability to hold alignment
- Trunk rotation

Start position

Seated, with knees bent in crook position

Instructions and teaching points

1. Inhale to prepare.
2. Exhale, engage abdominals and slide right leg out straight.
3. Inhale to prepare, maintaining abdominal connection and lengthening spine.
4. Exhale to cross the right leg over the left, placing the foot of the right leg on the floor by the side of the straight, left leg.
5. Inhale and hold position.
6. Exhale and lengthen the spine, maintaining connection of ribs and pelvis.
7. Twist the body towards the right, placing the right elbow against the outside of the right knee to ease the stretch further if flexibility allows (not if the spine collapses and the scapula placement is lost).
8. Keep the buttocks firmly placed on the floor.
9. Hold the stretch position and breathe laterally.
10. Return on an exhale.

Variations

- Perform sitting on a block for persons with less hamstring flexibility.
- Start with a smaller range of motion by not twisting the body around so far.
- Move progressively to a greater range of motion by twisting further around and using the arm to ease the leg further away from the direction in which the body is turning.

Ex. 5.18   Seated abductor stretch

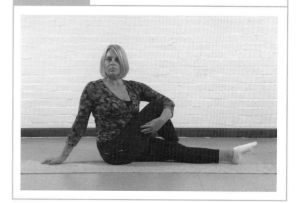

Exercise 5.19 Prone lying leg curl (all levels)

See Ex. 5.19

Purpose

- Develop awareness and felt connection between pelvic girdle and hip
- Pelvic stability
- Strengthen gluteal and hamstring muscles
- Actively lengthen quadriceps
- Trunk stability
- Ribcage placement
- Movement isolation

Start position

Prone lying, with hands resting under forehead

Instructions and teaching points

1. Inhale to prepare.
2. Exhale, engage abdominals, keep the tummy button lifted upwards (visualise an egg under the tummy button).
3. Maintaining placement of ribcage, extend and raise the leg back and upwards, curling the heel to the buttocks.
4. Inhale, lengthen and lower the leg to start position.
5. Maintain neutral alignment and take care not to press the weight on to the opposite leg.

Variations

- One leg at a time
- Alternate legs
- Both legs together with care!
- Could be performed in hands and knees position – one leg at a time

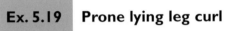

Ex. 5.19   **Prone lying leg curl**

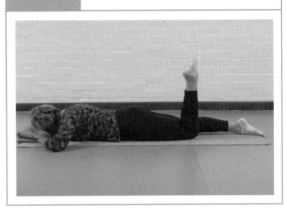

THE SHOULDER GIRDLE AND SHOULDER JOINT

6

Structure of the shoulder girdle

The shoulder girdle provides the connection between the arms and the spine. It is formed by the joining of the collarbones (clavicles) at the front, and shoulder blades (scapulae) at the back, on to the upper right and left sides of the skeleton (sternum and ribcage), with the arms (humerus) being the most distal connections (furthest away from centre) of the structure. The whole configuration can be visualised as having an American footballer's protective shoulder pads pulled on over the head (Hately-Aldous, 2005).

The *clavicles* are the long, thin, curved bones that run across the top of the chest horizontally from the sternum to the tip of the shoulder. They can be felt above the chest and just below the neck and can be observed in leaner individuals.

The *scapulae* are the triangular-shaped flat bones that partially cover the back of ribs 2 to 7. Along the top and back edge of the scapulae, there is a raised ridge that ends with a large bony process that can be felt at the top of the shoulder (the acromion process).

Note: To check positioning, slide the fingers down the side of the arm away from this tip (roughly 1 inch) to find the head of the humerus (shoulder joint). Rotating or twisting the arm inwards and outwards will cause the head of the humerus to rotate.

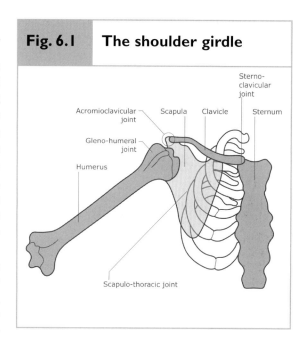

Fig. 6.1   The shoulder girdle

Sterno-clavicular joint

Acromioclavicular joint

Scapula

Clavicle

Sternum

Gleno-humeral joint

Humerus

Scapulo-thoracic joint

The functions of the shoulder girdle

The acromio-clavicular joint (AC joint)

This occurs where the collarbones meet the scapulae at the top, outer edge (lateral) of the shoulder (acromion process) to form a synovial joint (gliding). Sliding the fingers in towards the neck and away from the acromion process (roughly 1 inch) will find the acromio-clavicular joint.

The sterno-clavicular joint

This occurs where the collarbones join the sternum or breastbone (top and front) to form the synovial (saddle) joint. This joint has a cartilaginous disc that serves to absorb impact stress when falling and landing on an outstretched arm (which can cause 'jarring' of the shoulder). This joint is so strong that it is more likely that the bone (clavicle) will break from the jarring that occurs during such falls.

The joint actions and movements available at these aspects of the shoulder girdle include:

- Lifting the shoulders upwards towards the ears (elevation);
- Lowering the shoulders down away from the ears and drawing the scapulae down towards the buttocks (depression);
- Rounding the shoulders and shoulder girdle forwards in a hunching action (protraction);
- Opening the chest and shoulders by drawing the shoulder girdle backwards (retraction).

The scapulo-thoracic joint

This occurs where the scapulae meet the ribcage. The scapulae are able to slide over the ribcage during movements where the shoulders lift and lower. The movement that is available between the shoulder blades and the ribs is essential in maintaining mobility and stability of the shoulder girdle. Range of motion in this area will be affected by the range of movement available at both the acromio-clavicular and sterno-clavicular joints.

Restriction in range of movement at these joints (due to tightened and/or weakened muscles surrounding the structure) will reduce the range of movement available between the scapulae and the ribs and reduce stability. This may contribute to the scapulae being misaligned with the ribs, as in winging of the scapulae, whereby the inferior (lower) tip of the scapula and the medial part (inner border – closest to the spine) poke out and backwards.

The gleno-humeral or shoulder joint

This occurs where the head of the humerus joins the scapula just below the AC joint. The humerus fits into the shallow socket at the top and side (lateral) edge of the scapula – the *glenoid cavity*.

The shoulder joint is quite shallow, allowing the arm to hang down the side of the body when relaxed and to accomplish a large range of movement in many directions when specific muscles are activated. The movements available at the shoulder joint include:

- Raising the arm vertically upwards in front of the body (flexion and hyperflexion);
- Lowering the arm vertically down and behind the body (extension and hyperextension);
- Taking the arm out and away from the side of the body (abduction);
- Bringing the arm inwards in a sideways movement, across the front of the body (adduction);
- Twisting the arm inwards and outwards (medial and lateral rotation);
- A circular movement where the arm is taken in front of the body overhead and behind the body (circumduction);
- Hugging movements, where the arms are drawn horizontally in front of the body towards each other (horizontal flexion);
- Opening the arms horizontally away from each other and taking them backwards (horizontal extension).

Movements of the shoulder joint must be controlled and performed with correct technique to prevent injury, particularly when working in larger ranges of movement and/or using resistance or weight.

Muscles supporting and moving the shoulder girdle

Note: Refer to The major muscles diagrams on pp. 40–41 for the position of the different muscles.

There are many muscles that serve to mobilise (move) and stabilise the shoulder girdle and shoulder joint.

The *stabiliser muscles* include:
• The muscles that maintain the stability and position of the scapulae in relation to the ribcage, spine and pelvis during movement – serratus anterior, rhomboids, trapezius, levator scapulae, pectorals, latissimus dorsi);
• The muscles that help to keep the shoulder joint stable during movement. These are the rotator cuff muscles (infraspinatus, teres minor, subscapularis and supraspinatus).

The *mobiliser muscles* include:
• The muscles that move the shoulder (gleno-humeral) joint in the numerous directions listed above – latissimus dorsi, deltoids, pectorals, biceps and triceps.

Table 6.1	Trapezius
Description and muscle action	Large trapezium/kite-shaped muscle. Runs from the back of the skull, down the back of the neck, across the upper back to the shoulders and in between and slightly below the shoulder blades. Attaches to all thoracic vertebrae
Actions:	Upper (superior) fibres • Straighten/extend neck and keep head upright • Lift shoulder girdle Middle fibres • Draw back shoulder girdle • Adduct scapulae Lower (inferior) fibres • Draw shoulder girdle down – for example, when sliding the scapulae down towards the buttocks

Table 6.2	Rhomboids
• Rhomboid major • Rhomboid minor	
Description and muscle action	Short, rectangular muscle. Attaches on the inner (medial) edge of the scapula.
Actions:	• Stabilising the scapula • Assist middle fibres of trapezius to draw back (retract) the scapula • Assist adduction of the arm

Table 6.3	Serratus anterior
Description and muscle action	Attaches to the front of first eight ribs and the front, inner edge (anterior/medial border) of the scapula.
Actions:	• Draws the scapula forwards (protracts)

Table 6.4	Pectoralis minor
Description and muscle action	Thin muscle that lies underneath (deeper) pectoralis major. Runs outwards from the front of ribs 3-5 towards the shoulder and attaches to the top and front of the scapula (coracoid process).
Actions:	• Draws scapula forwards (protracts) • Elevates ribcage in forced breathing

Table 6.5	Levator scapulae
Description and muscle action	Strip of muscle that runs vertically at the rear side of the neck between C1 and C4 to the inner top border of the scapula.
Actions:	• Lifts the scapula • Bends neck to side (lateral flexion) • Assists trapezius and rhomboids to draw scapula inwards and upwards

Table 6.6	Deltoids
Description and muscle action	Thick, short muscle with three parts covering the top of the shoulder at the: front (anterior), centre (medial) and back (posterior). Attaches from the clavicle, acromion process and scapula to the humerus.
Actions:	Front (anterior) • Flexes and inwardly rotates arm Middle (medial) • Abducts the arm Back (posterior) • Extends the arm • Outwardly rotates the arm

Table 6.7	Pectoralis major
Description and muscle action	Broad band of muscle forming a 'fan' shape. Runs across the front right and left sides of the chest. Attaches from the clavicle, sternum and first six cartilages (ribs). Forms an aponeurosis with external oblique and attaches to the humerus.
Actions:	• Adducts the arm • Flexes the arm • Inwardly rotates the arm • Depresses the arm and shoulder

Table 6.8	Latissimus dorsi
Description and muscle action	Large, triangular muscle. Spans the right and left sides of the lower back and runs upwards towards the armpit (right and left sides). Attaches from the lower six thoracic vertebrae, lower (inferior) edge of scapula, lumbar vertebrae, thoracolumbar fascia, sacral vertebrae and iliac crest of pelvis to the humerus.
Actions:	• Extension of the arm • Adduction of the arm • Inward rotation of the arm • Keeps the lower scapula against the ribcage Used during powerful movements that pull the arm down (lat pull down, swimming) or pull the body up (chin-ups)

Table 6.9	Rotator cuff muscles
• Subscapularis • Supraspinatus	• Infraspinatus • Teres minor
Description and muscle action	Group of four short, broad muscles that attach from scapula to humerus.
Actions:	• Primary function to stabilise the shoulder (gleno-humeral) joint by holding the head of humerus into glenoid cavity and preventing dislocation of the shoulder when performing other movements of the arm • Three of the group rotate the shoulder. Prone to wear and tear (because of their stabilising role). Exert downward pull to counteract the opposing upward pull of the deltoids. Tendons can become compressed (impinged) by the bony parts of the shoulder joint, or they can tear/rupture. All movements of the shoulder joint should be performed carefully, but particular care should be taken with overhead activities involving rotational movement, such as throwing.

Table 6.9	Rotator cuff muscles (contd)
Subscapularis	Flat deep muscle band that cannot be felt/palpated. Front surface of scapula attaching to humerus. Positioned next to serratus anterior.
Actions	• Inward (medial) rotation • Assists with flexion, extension, adduction and abduction (Stone and Stone, 1990) • Stabilises shoulder joint
Supraspinatus	Top of the scapula, deep to the deltoid; cannot be felt/palpated.
Actions	• Assists deltoid with abduction (weak) • Prevents downwards dislocation of shoulder when carrying heavy bags Stone and Stone (1990); Thompson (1989)
Infraspinatus	Flat muscle band at back of scapula to humerus. Can be felt/palpated between humerus and scapula, below posterior deltoid (Thompson, 1989). Deep position, underneath trapezius.
Actions	• Rotates the arm outwards (laterally) • Lower part adducts the arm • Horizontal extension and extension of shoulder • Stabilises shoulder joint Stone and Stone (1990); Thompson (1989)
Teres minor	Thin muscle. Border of scapula to humerus. Can be felt/palpated between humerus and scapula, below posterior deltoid (Thompson, 1989).
Actions	• Rotates the arm outwards (laterally) • Horizontal extension and extension of shoulder • Stabilises shoulder joint

Theory to practice – application

The shoulder girdle is a complex structure and its functioning will be affected by many factors. These may include:

- The alignment of the spine and position of the head
- The tension (overactivity/inactivity) of the surrounding muscles
- The method of breathing we use most often (breathing is discussed further in chapter 8)
- The stability of the pelvis and core muscles in this region
- The functioning and strength of lower limbs
- Our ability to relax (body and mind)
- Our emotional state and thinking processes.

It is quite common for the muscles of the upper shoulder and shoulder girdle (upper fibres of trapezius and levator scapulae) to be overused and as a consequence become tighter and shortened. The muscles below the scapulae (lower and middle fibres of trapezius) are often weaker and lengthened.

In Pilates, the positioning and movement of the shoulder girdle is made a focus of attention. For example, we might notice:

- The position of the shoulders in relation to the ears
- How the shoulders move when the arm moves
- Any changes in the position of the ribcage and the head when the shoulders move
- How the weight distribution in the lower body is experienced when the arm moves.

For many people, most of the time, all this happens without them being aware of it. Consequently, movements of the shoulder are clumsy and poorly aligned, controlled and performed. Lack of awareness will not serve to improve the dysfunctions of movement. But awareness can help to improve both these dysfunctions and stability and mobility.

With regard to emotional state, from a practical perspective we literally have to move the shoulder girdle to hug, hold and caress. The experience of hugging and being hugged is for many a relieving and releasing experience, which may reflect a willingness to be receptive to both giving and receiving.

The positioning of the shoulder girdle can reflect our feelings. When we are receptive, confident and feeling positive, there will be more openness and expansion. When we are feeling sad or stressed, carrying tension, lacking confidence, grieving and so on, there will be a closed, sinking and hunched appearance. The mind and emotions are explored further in chapter 9.

Modified exercises

Exercise 6.1 Lying arm floats – front (all levels)

See Ex. 6.1

Purpose

- Shoulder joint mobility
- Develop awareness and felt connection between shoulder girdle and arm movements
- Shoulder stability
- Ribcage placement
- Movement isolation

Start position

Supine crook lying, with arms at side of body

Instructions and teaching points

1. Inhale to prepare, ensuring shoulders are relaxed down away from the ears. Feel the shoulder blades connecting with the floor.
2. Exhale, engage abdominals and draw scapula down, keeping ribcage relaxed and floating the arm upwards to a position level with the shoulders.
3. Inhale to lower back down.

Variations

- One arm at a time
- Alternate arms
- Both arms together

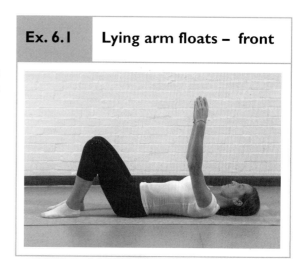

Ex. 6.1   **Lying arm floats – front**

Exercise 6.2 Standing arm floats – front (all levels)

See Ex. 6.2

Ex. 6.2	Standing arm floats – front

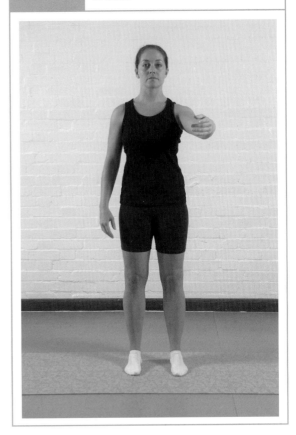

Purpose

- Shoulder joint mobility
- Develop awareness and felt connection between shoulder girdle and arm movements
- Shoulder stability
- Ribcage placement
- Movement isolation

Start position

Standing posture, with arms at side of body

Instructions and teaching points

1. Inhale to prepare, ensuring shoulders are relaxed down away from the ears (in a lying position).
2. Feel the shoulder blades sliding down towards the buttocks and the chest opening.
3. Exhale and engage abdominals, draw scapula down towards buttocks and float the arm upwards to a position level with the shoulders.
4. Keep the ribcage relaxed and not protruding forwards.
5. Keep the chest open – visualise a rod through the sides of the shoulder.
6. Inhale to lower back down.

Variations

- One arm at a time
- Alternate arms
- Both arms together
- Balance on one leg to perform
- Can combine with heel raises

Exercise 6.3 Lying overhead arm floats – front (levels 2/3/4)

See Ex. 6.3

Purpose

- Shoulder joint mobility
- Develop awareness and felt connection between shoulder girdle and arm movements
- Shoulder stability
- Trunk stability
- Ribcage placement
- Movement isolation
- Active lengthening of anterior deltoid as arm lowers to floor

Start position

Supine crook lying, with arms raised to shoulder height

Instructions and teaching points

1. Inhale to prepare, ensuring shoulders are relaxed down away from the ears (in a lying position).
2. Feel the shoulder blades connecting with the floor and imagine them sliding down towards the buttocks.
3. Exhale and engage abdominals.
4. Keep the ribcage aligned (not protruding upwards), head aligned (not tilting back) and float the arms towards the floor.
5. Inhale at bottom.
6. Exhale and engage abdominals, keeping ribcage connected, and lift back to start position.
7. Restrict range of motion to what feels comfortable (persons with instability in this area should ensure they maintain control to avoid clunking sensations while lowering arms.

Variations

- One arm at a time
- Alternate arms
- Both arms together

Ex. 6.3	Lying overhead arm floats – front

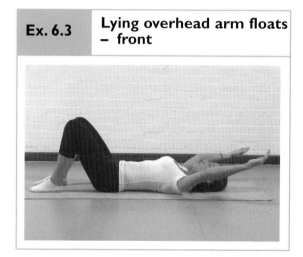

Exercise 6.4 Standing overhead arm floats – front (levels 2/3/4)

See Ex. 6.4

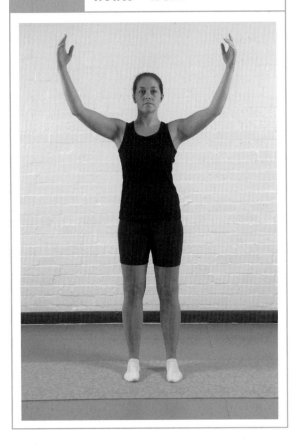

Ex. 6.4	**Standing overhead arm floats – front**

Purpose

- Shoulder joint mobility
- Develop awareness and felt connection between shoulder girdle and arm movements
- Shoulder stability
- Trunk stability
- Ribcage placement
- Movement isolation

Start position

Standing posture, with arms raised to chest height

Instructions and teaching points

1. Inhale to prepare, ensuring shoulders are relaxed down away from the ears.
2. Visualise the shoulder blades sliding down towards the buttocks and open the chest (as if there were a rod through the shoulders).
3. Exhale and engage abdominals.
4. Keep ribcage relaxed and aligned (not poking forwards or lifting), floating the arm overhead.
5. Inhale at the lower.
6. Ensure the shoulders do not lift towards the ears or protract forwards.

Variations

- One arm at a time
- Alternate arms
- Both arms together
- Standing on one leg
- Combine with heel raises
- Perform seated on stability ball

Exercise 6.5 Lying lateral arm slides (all levels)

See Ex. 6.5

Purpose

- Shoulder joint mobility
- Develop awareness and felt connection between shoulder girdle and arm movements
- Shoulder stability
- Trunk stability
- Ribcage placement
- Movement isolation

Start position

Supine crook lying, with arms at side of the body, palms face up

Instructions and teaching points

1. Inhale to prepare, ensuring shoulders are relaxed down away from the ears (in a lying position).
2. Feel the shoulder blades connecting with the floor and imagine them sliding down towards the buttocks.
3. Exhale and engage abdominals.
4. Keep the ribcage aligned (not protruding upwards) and head aligned (not tilting back).
5. Slide the arm out to the side of the body to shoulder height.

6. Inhale at the top.
7. Exhale, engage abdominals, keeping ribcage connected, and lengthen back to start position.

Variations

- One arm at a time
- Alternate arms
- Both arms together
- Can increase range of motion and take arm over head – keeping shoulders away from ears and minimising movement of the scapulae

Ex. 6.5	Lying lateral arm slides

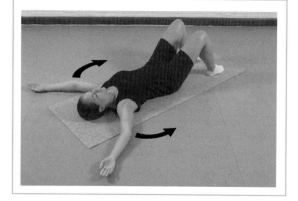

Exercise 6.6 Standing lateral arm raise (all levels)

See Ex. 6.6

Ex. 6.6	Standing lateral arm raise

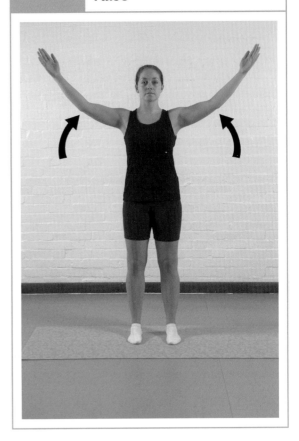

Purpose

- Shoulder joint mobility
- Develop awareness and felt connection between shoulder girdle and arm movements
- Shoulder stability
- Trunk stability
- Ribcage placement
- Movement isolation

Start position

Standing with the arms at side of the body, palms face forwards

Instructions and teaching points

1. Inhale to prepare, ensuring shoulders are relaxed down away from the ears (in a lying position).
2. Feel the shoulder blades sliding down towards the buttocks.
3. Exhale and engage abdominals.
4. Keep the ribcage aligned (not protruding upwards) and the head aligned (not tilting back).
5. Raise the arm out to the side of the body to shoulder height.
6. Keep drawing the shoulder blades down and keep the chest open.
7. Inhale to lower arm.

Variations

- One arm at a time.
- Alternate arms
- Both arms together
- Can increase range of motion and take arm over head – keeping shoulders away from ears and ensuring minimal movement of the scapulae
- Perform seated on a stability ball

Exercise 6.7 Lying shoulder shrugs (all levels)

See Ex. 6.7

Purpose

- Develop awareness and felt connection between shoulder girdle and arm movements
- Shoulder girdle mobility
- Lengthen muscles between spine and scapulae
- Trunk stability
- Ribcage placement
- Movement isolation

Start position

Supine crook lying, with arms raised to shoulder height

Instructions and teaching points

1. Inhale to prepare, ensuring shoulders are relaxed down away from the ears (in a lying position).
2. Feel the shoulder blades connecting with the floor and imagine them sliding down towards the buttocks.
3. Exhale and engage abdominals.
4. Keep the ribcage aligned (not protruding upwards) and head aligned (not tilting back).
5. Reach the arm up as if to grab an object slightly above fingertips. The scapulae will slide outwards.
6. Inhale to lower.

Variations

- One arm at a time
- Alternate arms
- Both arms together

Ex. 6.7	Lying shoulder shrugs

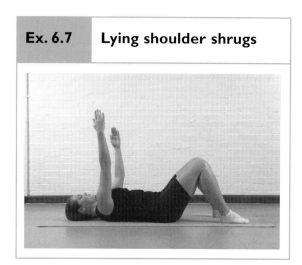

Exercise 6.8 Hands and knees cat peddle (all levels)

See Ex. 6.8

Purpose

- Develop awareness and felt connection between shoulder girdle and arm movements
- Shoulder stability
- Strengthen muscles between shoulder blades
- Trunk stability
- Ribcage placement
- Movement isolation
- Develop balance

Start position

Hands and knees

Instructions and teaching points

1. Inhale to prepare. Lengthen shoulders down away from ears and slide shoulder blades towards buttocks.
2. Exhale and engage abdominals.
3. Strengthen connection at shoulder blades (not dropping forwards) and raise the hand slightly away from the floor.
4. Inhale to lower hand.

Variations

- Just getting into a correct hands and knees position, and holding it, may be a sufficient starting point for someone with instability around the scapulae

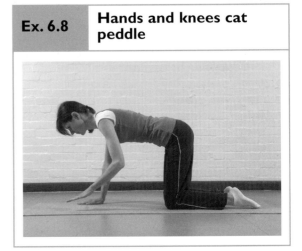

| Ex. 6.8 | **Hands and knees cat peddle** |

Exercise 6.9 Hands and knees arm reach (levels 2/3/4)

See Ex. 6.9

Purpose

- Develop awareness and felt connection between shoulder girdle and arm movements
- Shoulder stability
- Strengthen muscles between shoulder blades
- Trunk stability
- Ribcage placement
- Movement isolation
- Develop balance

Start position

Hands and knees

Instructions and teaching points

1. Inhale to prepare. Lengthen shoulders down away from ears and slide shoulder blades towards buttocks.
2. Exhale and engage abdominals.
3. Strengthen connection at shoulder blades (not dropping forwards) and reach forwards without dropping shoulders or scrunching them to ears. The arm should reach to a point on the floor in front of the body.
4. Inhale to lower arm.

Variations

- Can be progressed by reaching forwards and lifting the arm upwards towards the ceiling – provided ribcage placement is not compromised (Ex. 6.9b).
- Can be progressed further by combining with leg raise to rear (Ex. 6.9b).

Ex. 6.9a | **Hands and knees arm reach**

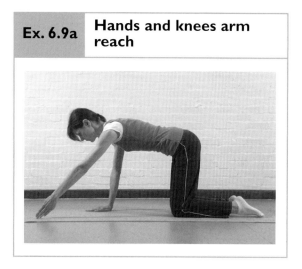

Ex. 6.9b | **Variations**

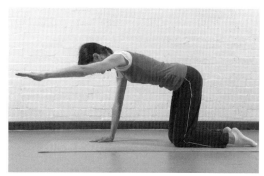

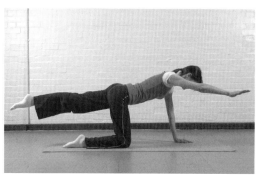

Exercise 6.10 Supine lying chest stretch (all levels)

See Ex. 6.10

Purpose

- Develop awareness and felt connection between shoulder girdle and arm movements
- Lengthen and stretch muscles at front of chest and shoulder (pectorals and anterior deltoid)
- Ribcage placement

Start position

Supine crook lying

Instructions and teaching points

1. Inhale to prepare.
2. Keep shoulders relaxed and down away from the ears.
3. Exhale, engage abdominals and raise arms to the side of the body in a crucifix position, keeping shoulders away from the ears.
4. Ensure ribcage does not rise.
5. Hold the position breathing laterally.
6. Return on an exhale.

Variations

- Bend the elbows at right angles in same position described above
- Place a block underneath elbows and wrists for persons with less flexibility

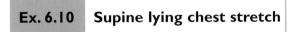

Ex. 6.10 **Supine lying chest stretch**

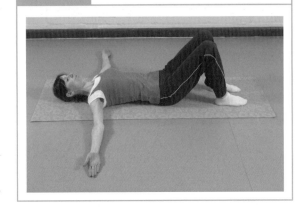

Exercise 6.11 Prone lying dart (all levels)

See Ex. 6.11

Purpose

- Strengthen muscles between the shoulder blades
- Develop awareness and connection between the shoulder girdle and arms
- Develop awareness of alignment of neck and head
- Pelvic stability
- Active lengthening of anterior deltoid and pectoral muscles
- Maintain connection between ribcage and pelvis

Start position

Prone lying, with hands alongside body and palms facing upwards

Instructions and teaching points

1. Inhale to prepare.
2. Exhale, engage abdominals and visualise tummy lifting away from the floor (not moving pelvis).
3. Raise shoulders slightly towards the ceiling (retract) and slide them towards buttocks (depression).
4. At the same time, rotate the palm to face the thigh, so that the shoulder externally rotates.
5. Inhale to return.

Variations

- Progress by allowing upper body to lift slightly from floor without tilting head
- Place hands in a W position, with the elbows bent at 90 degrees out to the side of the body, elbows positioned slightly lower than the armpits
- Progress to breaststroke, which combines W position raise with dart

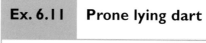

Ex. 6.11   Prone lying dart

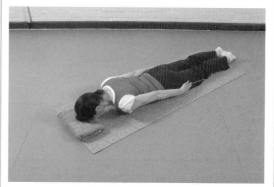

Exercise 6.12 Prone lying breaststroke swim (levels 2/3/4)

See 6.12

Purpose

- Strengthen muscles between the shoulder blades
- Develop awareness and connection between the shoulder girdle and arms
- Develop awareness of alignment of neck and head
- Pelvic stability
- Active lengthening of anterior deltoid and pectoral muscles
- Maintain connection between ribcage and pelvis
- Shoulder mobility

Start position

Prone lying with hands in W position. Elbows bent at 90 degrees out to the side of the body, elbows positioned slightly lower than the armpits.

Instructions and teaching points

1. Inhale to prepare.
2. Exhale, engage abdominals and visualise tummy lifting away from the floor (not moving pelvis).
3. Raise shoulders slightly towards the ceiling (retract) and slide them towards buttocks (depression).
4. At the same time, raise the hands and elbows slightly from the floor.
5. Inhale and maintain position.
6. Exhale and reach arms forwards over head (without scrunching shoulders to ears).
7. When arms are fully extended, rotate the shoulder outwards so the palm turns out and sweep the hands out in a breaststroke swimming action to end in dart position.
8. Inhale to return to W position.
9. Watch that the shoulders do not rotate forwards.

Variations

- Progress to raising the upper body as the arms lift
- Vary the breathing: inhale to prepare, exhale for raise and breaststroke, inhale to return to W

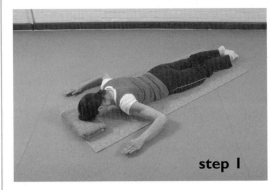
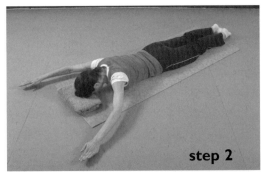
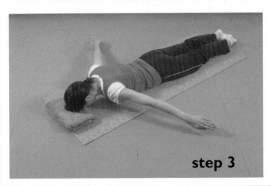

Ex. 6.12	Prone lying breaststroke swim

step 1

step 2

step 3

Exercise 6.13 Hands and knees to plank (levels 2/3/4)

See Ex. 6.13

Purpose

- Develop awareness and felt connection between shoulder girdle and arm movements
- Shoulder and pelvic stability
- Strengthen muscles between shoulder blades
- Ribcage placement
- Upper body strength

Start position

Hands and knees

Instructions and teaching points

1. Inhale to prepare.
2. Lengthen shoulders down away from ears and slide shoulder blades towards buttocks.
3. Exhale, engage abdominals and strengthen connection at shoulder blades (not dropping forwards).
4. Slide one leg back to extended position.
5. Inhale and hold position.
6. Exhale, maintain abdominal engagement and slide other leg back (balls of both feet now resting on the floor).
7. Hold position and maintain lateral breathing.
8. Return on an exhale.

Variations

- Rear leg raises from hands and knees need to be performed adequately before progressing to plank. You must also be able to hold a stable hands and knees position.
- Progressions can be to include leg raises from the plank position.

Ex. 6.13a **¾ plank elbow variation**

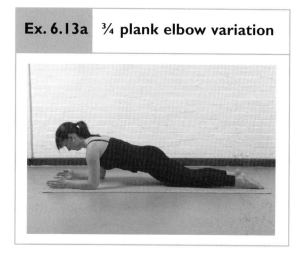

Ex. 6.13b **Full plank**

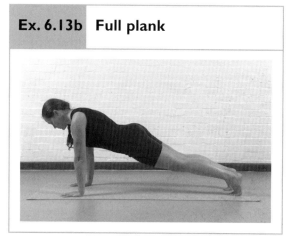

Ex. 6.13c **Full plank, elbow variation**

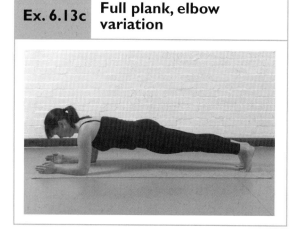

Exercise 6.14 Hands and knees press-up (levels 2/3/4)

See Ex. 6.14

Purpose

- Develop awareness and felt connection between shoulder girdle and arm movements
- Shoulder and pelvic stability
- Strengthen pectoral, anterior deltoid and tricep muscles
- Strength and stability for muscles between shoulder blades
- Ribcage placement

Start position

Hands and knees

Instructions and teaching points

1. Inhale to prepare. Lengthen shoulders down away from ears and slide shoulder blades towards buttocks.
2. Exhale, engage abdominals and strengthen connection at shoulder blades (not dropping forwards).
3. Bend elbows backwards (keeping them into sides of the body) so that head lowers in between the hands (keep neck aligned).
4. Inhale and hold position.
5. Exhale, maintain abdominal engagement and press up to full extension at elbows.

Variations

- Vary breath to single time – inhale and lower, exhale and lift. Three-quarter position, where front of thigh rests on floor
- Full position, starting from plank (6.14b)

Ex. 6.14a | **Hands and knees press-up**

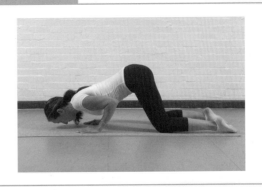

Ex. 6.14b | **¾ press-up**

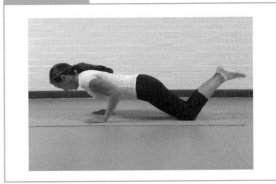

Ex. 6.14c | **Full press-up**

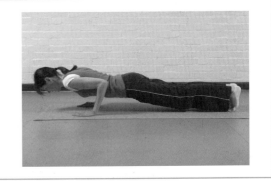

POSTURE AND POSTURE TYPES

7

Posture is used to describe the way the body is positioned and carried when still/static (standing and sitting) or moving/dynamic (walking and running). Optimal posture is that which enables gravitational forces to be spread equally throughout the body, promoting maximal movement efficiency (no unnecessary muscle or joint activity) and minimal stress (wear and tear) on the body (tissues and inner organs).

to alleviate a build up of muscular tension, and they can also enhance the functioning of inner organs (for example, the diaphragm). Standing and moving with correct posture gives the impression of greater confidence and indeed walking with upright posture can increase personal confidence. Open posture is expansive. Hunched over posture gives the appearance of closing in on oneself.

Why is correct posture important?

Postural misalignment can affect the functioning of our inner organs. For example, allowing the mid section to rest continuously in a slumped position can affect the movement of the diaphragm, the muscle that assists with breathing.

Poor posture that is maintained and uncorrected for long periods of time can also lead to permanent postural problems, for example hunched back (kyphosis), which can contribute to the risk of falls in later life, or hollow back posture (lordosis), which can contribute to back pain.

Prolonged muscle imbalance by holding an incorrect posture will also lead to increased muscle tension and tightness in some muscles and a lack of strength or lengthening in opposing muscles.

Exercises to open and align posture can help

Centre of gravity, stability and balance

The centre of gravity is positioned in the pelvic region and passes between the hips and forwards of the sacrum. The body is considered to be balanced when the centre of gravity falls within its base of support. For example, when standing the base of support will be the position of the feet. When on hands and knees, the base of support will be the hands and knees. The relationship between the centre of gravity and balance and stability will be determined by the exercise position and the stability of the base of support. For example, standing on one leg will offer less stability than would standing with the weight distributed through both feet.

Balance is assisted and maintained by visual cues (the eyes), the sense of equilibrium monitored by the middle ear and the positioning and the proprioceptors in the joints and muscles.

When standing upright, the body is relatively unstable because the centre of gravity is higher and the base of support (feet) is smaller. When lying on the back (supine), the base of support is wide and the centre of gravity is low, thus lying is a more stable position.

Assessment of posture – observation from the side

The plumb line posture provides a standard from which deviations can be measured. When observing the body from the side, the plumb line runs down the centre of the side of the body from:

- The crown of the head
- Ear lobe (position of an earring)
- Cervical vertebrae
- Shoulder joint (head of humerus)
- Lumbar vertebrae
- ASIS and PSIS of pelvis level
- Hip joint (greater trochanter)
- Knee joint (slightly in front of axis where knee bends)
- Ankle joint (slightly in front of malleolus – prominent bone at side of ankle).

Fig. 7.1	Plumb line

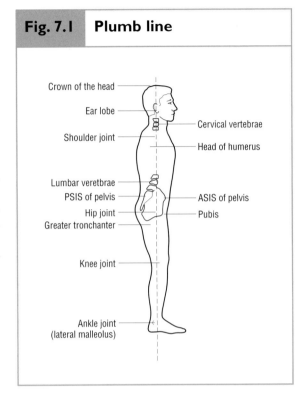

Crown of the head
Ear lobe
Cervical vertebrae
Shoulder joint
Head of humerus
Lumbar veretbrae
PSIS of pelvis
ASIS of pelvis
Hip joint
Pubis
Greater tronchanter
Knee joint
Ankle joint
(lateral malleolus)

Deviations to alignment can be at any of these points and will give an indication of what posture type an individual presents with. This can also provide a guide for where imbalances between muscle strength and flexibility exist.

Table 7.1	
Body part	Optimal alignment
Neck	Upright and erect – no marked chin poking
Chest	Breastbone furthest forward – no marked depression or flattening of chest
Shoulders	Central – no marked protrusion of shoulder blades at rear
Upper back	Normal rounding – no marked rounding
Trunk	Upright – no marked backward sway
Abdomen	Flat – no marked protrusion or sagging of the abdominals
Lower back	Natural curve – no marked hollowing

Adapted version of New York Posture Rating test (in Davis Kimmet Auty, 1996).

Assessment of posture – observation from the back

Table 7.2	
Body part	Optimal alignment
Head	Aligned centrally and not leaning to either right or left side
Shoulders	Level with each other, ideally with a space between the shoulders and ears, without one shoulder being positioned higher than the other
Spine	Straight – no apparent C or S curves
Shoulder blades (scapulae)	Lower points of scapulae should be level. The inner (medial) borders should be vertical and there should be equal space between the medial borders and thoracic vertebrae on both sides. The positioning/stability of the scapulae can also be checked from an all fours position to observe whether the scapulae lie flat or protrude away from ribs. The stability of the scapulae can be felt by placing the hand on the scapula and abducting the arm. During the first 30 degrees of abduction there should be no movement. Between 30 and 90 degrees, the scapula should begin to rotate upwards and the inferior tip move to the side. Beyond 90 degrees, the scapula moves laterally around the ribcage.
Hips	Level – no marked difference between height of hips and height of pelvis
Waist	There should be equal skin creases at the waist
Buttocks	The underneath of the buttock cheeks should be level, without one buttock dropping lower than the other
Knee creases	The level of the knee creases should be equal
Calf muscle	The bulk of the calf muscles should be equal
Foot position	Feet point straight forwards – no marked outward pointing of feet or rolling inwards of ankles
Feet arches	There should be an equal arching of the feet (not flat or excessively arched)

Adapted version of New York Posture Rating test (in Davis Kimmet Auty, 1996)

The body is rarely purely symmetrical or balanced equally between right and left sides. In fact, a little asymmetry or mild imbalance is normal for most people (Latey, 2001). However, when the asymmetry is pronounced enough to affect functioning or balance and causes discomfort, for example scoliosis, this should be referred for treatment and management by a physiotherapist.

Posture assessment of the shoulder girdle

Table 7.3

General appearance when standing upright	Should be flat against ribcage and not protruding back
General appearance when weight is on all fours	Should be flat against ribcage and not protruding back
Distance between medial border of scapula and spine	Ideally, equal distance both sides, equivalent to width of middle three fingers of the person's hand
Alignment of medial border	Should be vertical from top to bottom
Position of arm	Arm should be positioned in line with plumb line, not forward
Position of scapulae during abduction when standing	First 30 degrees should remain flat against ribcage without movement. From 30 to 90 degrees slight upward rotation. Humerus rotates laterally so that inner elbow faces upwards. From 90 degrees thoracic spine flattens. Sternum lifts and scapulae slide around ribcage when humerus is level with ear.
Position of scapulae on all fours and raising hand (cat peddle)	Should remain flat against ribcage

Factors affecting posture

Many factors may contribute to changes of postural misalignment, whereby one set of muscles may become less active and/or lengthened and another set of muscles may become overactive and/or shortened, resulting in the spine and structures being pulled away from plumb line alignment. These factors include:

Fashion

Wearing shoes with high heels or carrying backpacks will throw the centre of gravity out of balance and the body will need to compensate alignment to maintain balance. Carrying bags on the same shoulder, or always using the same arm to lift heavy suitcases, will contribute to imbalances between right and left sides.

Work/school

Lifestyles that demand repetitive sustaining of the same sedentary positions, such as driving, operating a checkout or working with a computer, will contribute to muscle imbalances. Poor positioning or incorrect height of desks and chairs will also affect alignment, as indeed will the way we choose to sit at our desks and in our chairs.

Excessive usage of sedentary games (such as computer games) will also reduce activity levels and encourage sedentary patterns. Spending too much time watching TV or DVDs on a comfortable couch, and lying or sitting in slumped positions, will also have an effect on alignment.

In addition, the way in which we travel to work will affect posture. Imagine standing on a tube train for 45 minutes, with one arm raised above the head holding on to a strap attached to the ceiling to assist balance. In this position, the muscles of the upper back and neck will be shortening on one side of the body, leading to all sorts imbalances if not taken into considered and rectified.

Emotions

Lack of confidence, low self-esteem, stress or depression can all affect posture. For example, persons who lack confidence or who are feeling depressed may have a tendency to walk looking downwards towards the floor, avoiding eye contact with others. Repetitive looking down when walking will contribute to changes of posture, whereby the head tilts forwards, the shoulders round over and, ultimately, a kyphotic posture develops. (This posture can increase the risk of falls in older populations.)

Teenage girls with breasts developing earlier than those of the rest of their peers may find this threatening to their confidence and could start rounding their shoulders to hide the development. In addition, teenagers who are sensitive about being taller than their peers may also slouch to match the height of the peer group and not stand out.

Sport

Most sporting activities emphasise the predominant use of particular muscles, which notoriously creates some imbalance. Racquet sports and golf may develop muscles on one side of the body more than the other. Cycling for long distances may promote shortening of the hip flexor and hamstring muscles. Games such as football and rugby tend to demand greater attention to some components of fitness (strength and endurance, cardiovascular, speed, agility) at the expense of other components (flexibility), which again lead to imbalances. Breaststroke swimming may contribute to rounding of the shoulders. Gymnastics and dance may contribute to lordosis. Ideally, sports coaches will be aware of the potential for these imbalances and accommodate these within the training.

Inactivity

Lack of use will contribute to atrophy (decrease in muscle and strength). Untrained muscles are less able to function effectively against the forces of gravity.

Environment

Walking or running on uneven terrain can promote imbalance between the strength of muscles on one side of the body. Exercising in a cold environment may cause the posture to close in and hunch, in an attempt to keep huddled and warm. Likewise, walking outside in cold weather can cause a lifting of the shoulders and hunching of the upper spine to close in and keep warm.

Poorly designed furniture can also contribute to poor posture and alignment. Chairs that have C-shaped backs can promote C-shaped alignment of the spine.

Genetics/hereditary conditions

Family history can account for a specific posture problem. Scoliosis, for example, may be inherited. In addition, some children may copy posture and walking patterns from their parents or guardians.

Medical

Soft tissue injuries (strains and sprains), dislocations and bone fractures will limit functioning and movement until healing is complete. During this time, imbalances can occur. Changes in health due to more serious medical conditions (for example, heart attacks, angina) may promote a reduction in activity levels (because of fear of bringing on another attack). An increased sedentary lifestyle will affect posture.

Age

Anatomical changes that occur during the growth spurts of puberty (along with raised hormone levels) will contribute to all sorts of physical and emotional changes in teenagers that can affect their posture. Changes in bone density that occur through the ageing process (osteoporosis) will also have an impact on posture.

Physical disabilities

Individuals with hearing or sight limitations may over exaggerate some aspects of posture (head tilting or poking). The eyes and ears play an essential role in assisting balance and any minor (or major) disability will have an impact on posture.

Posture types

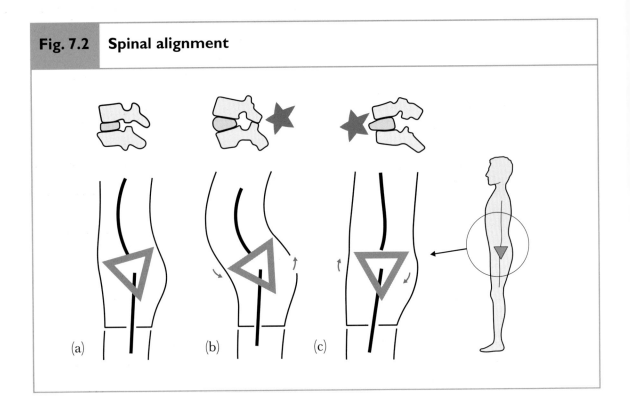

Fig. 7.2 Spinal alignment

Illustration (a) shows the neutral pelvic position.

Illustration (b) shows an anterior or forward pelvic tilt, providing the hollowing of the lower back observable in a lordotic curvature of the lumbar spine.

Illustration (c) shows a posterior tilt of the pelvis, which gives the lower back a flattened appearance, as in a flat back posture type.

Lordotic posture – lordosis

Fig. 7.3 Lordosis

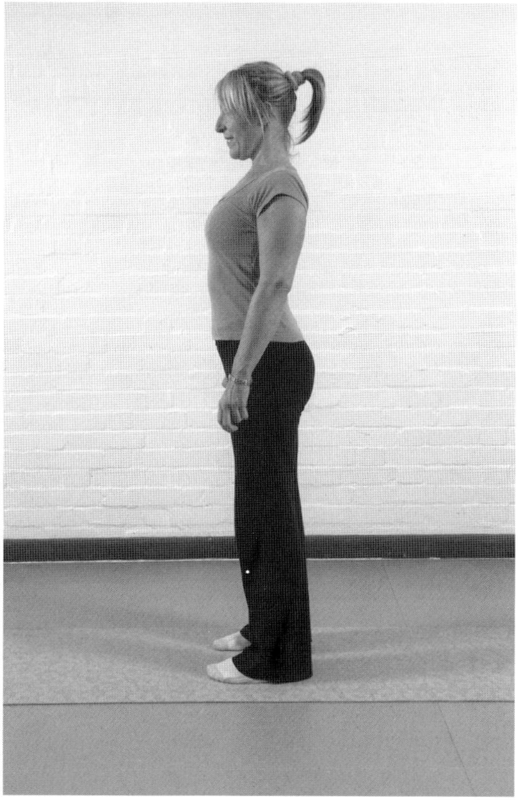

Lordosis is an exaggerated curve in the lumbar region of the spine. It can give the appearance of a deeper than normal hollow of the lower back. In this posture type, the anterior superior iliac spine (ASIS) is tilted forwards (anteriorly) and is lower than the posterior superior iliac spine (PSIS), creating an increased curvature of the lumbar spine.

Lordosis occurs when the abdominal and gluteal muscles are lengthened and the hip flexor and back extensors are shortened. Increased lumbar lordosis can give rise to compression of the facet joints in this region, causing pain and stiffness, which can further contribute to tightening of the hamstring muscles. However, it should be noted that tilting of the pelvis draws the hamstring into a lengthened rather than shortened position.

Summary of observable features of lordotic posture

Anterior tilt of the pelvis (ASIS lower than PSIS);

Lengthened and usually weaker rectus abdominis and external oblique muscles;

Gluteas maximus and medius are usually weaker, less active and lengthened;

Hamstrings may be tight, often overactive and working when they shouldn't (instead of gluteals), but not necessarily shortened;

Hip is in a flexed position;

Hip flexors are shortened;

Stiffness in lumbar spine;

Increased curve of lumbar spine – hyperextension;

Back extensors are shortened and tight;

Adductor muscle may be tight in response to forward flexed position of hip.

Lifestyle factors that may contribute to lordotic posture

Pregnancy, with the increasing baby weight lengthening and weakening the abdominals and shortening the back muscles;

High levels of body fat in the abdominal region;

Genetics – some people of African and Caribbean origin have a naturally deeper lordotic curve;

Gymnasts and dancers are prone to lordosis due to repetitive hyperextension of the lumbar spine required by some positions.

Recommendations to manage and improve lordotic posture

Strengthen and shorten the superficial abdominal muscles (rectus abdominis, external obliques);

Develop flexibility of the deeper and superficial back extensors (multifidus and erector spinae);

Develop flexibility of the hip flexor and adductor muscles;

Stretch the hamstring muscles;

Strengthen the deeper abdominals to hold a neutral pelvic position when seated and standing;

Strengthen and activate the gluteal muscles;

Mobility and flexion exercises for the lumbar spine.

Movements to limit lordotic posture

Hyperextension of the spine;

In some cases you might you want to include thoracic extension, but restrict lumber extension.

Recommended exercises

- Modified seated roll back – 'c' curve (4.5)
- Seated spine twists (4.1)
- All fours cat peddle (6.8)
- Pelvic tilts (4.2)
- Shoulder bridge (4.3)
- Supine heel raise (5.2)
- Supine knee raise (5.3)
- Supine foot dip from table top (5.4)
- Curl-up (4.7)
- Arm float variations (6.1-6.6)
- Hip flexor stretch (5.16/5.17)
- Hamstring stretch (5.12/5.15)
- Child pose/shell stretch (4.10)
- Supine lower back release (4.11)
- Cat stretch (rounding) (4.12)

Flat back posture

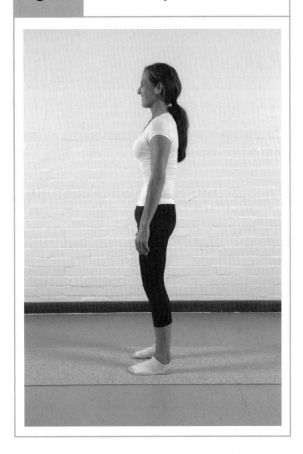

Fig. 7.4	Flat back posture

In this posture type the lumbar curve is reduced, giving a flattened appearance to the lower spine. There is a lack of mobility in the lumbar area.

Summary of observable features of flat back posture

Head may be forward of the plumb line (neck flexors weak);

Thoracic spine may be rounded at the top and flatter lower down;

Distinctive loss of lumbar curve and flattening of lower back;

Posterior tilt of pelvis (PSIS lower than ASIS);

Stiffness in lumbar spine;

Tightened/shortened rectus abdominis, especially upper fibres;

Tightened hamstrings, pulling pelvis down and back;

Hip flexors are lengthened and weaker;

Knee joints may be hyperextended, but can also be held in a flexed position.

Lifestyle factors that may contribute to flat back posture

Prolonged sitting at a desk in an incorrect position;

Prolonged driving in an incorrect position;

Any activity (or lack of) that contributes to poor core stability (sedentary lifestyle);

Stiffness in the lower back;

Performing excessive amounts of sit-ups with back pressing down to floor.

Recommendations to manage and improve flat back posture

Teach correct standing and sitting posture;

Teach correct lifting techniques (dead lift);

Promote mobility in the lumbar spine;

Strengthen the core abdominal muscles to assist maintenance of a neutral pelvic position;

Promote spine mobility, especially extension of the lumbar spine;

Stretch the hamstrings;

Strengthen and shorten the hip flexors (if there is posterior tilt);

Stretch the rectus abdominis.

Recommended exercises

- Modified seated roll back – 'c' curve (4.5)
- Prone lying leg raise (5.8)
- Gluteal bracing (5.9)
- Hands and knees leg extension (5.5)
- Shoulder bridge (4.3)
- Supine heel raise (5.2) and from standing
- Supine foot dip from table top (5.4)
- Modified standing roll down (4.4)
- Curl-up (4.7)
- Prone lying dart (6.11)
- Prone lying breaststroke swim (6.12)
- Arm float variations (6.1-6.6)
- Hip flexor stretch (5.16/5.17)
- Hamstring stretch (5.12/5.15)
- Child pose/shell stretch (4.10)
- Supine lower back release (4.11)
- Cat stretch (4.12)

Kyphotic posture – kyphosis

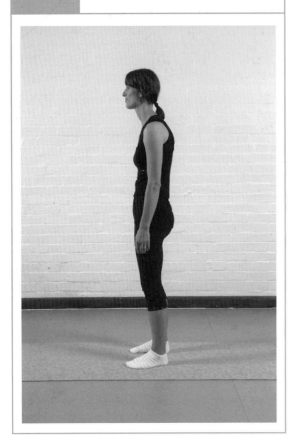

Fig. 7.5	Kyphosis

This is an exaggerated curvature in the thoracic region. It can give someone a hunched over and round-shouldered look.

Kyphosis occurs as a result of shortening of the muscles that protract the shoulder girdle (draw it forwards) – the pectoral muscles of the chest – and a lengthening of the muscles that retract the shoulder girdle (draw it backwards) – the trapezius and rhomboids. As the shoulders round forwards, away from the desired plumb line posture, they pull the thoracic spine forwards into a flexed (bent) forwards position). The weight of the arms adds weight, which increases the forward pull on the thoracic spine and causes the scapulae to slide round the ribcage, restricting the movement available at both the shoulder joint and the shoulder girdle.

Summary of observable features of kyphotic posture

Head and chin poking forwards;
Cervical spine is in hyperextension;
Upper trapezius is overactive and shortened;
Scapulae are abducted away from the ribcage;
Thoracic spine is in hyperflexion;
Less mobility of thoracic spine;
Thoracic back extensors are lengthened;
Pectoral muscles are shortened and tight;
Intercostal muscles are shortened;
Rectus abdominis is tight;
Lower trapezius and rhomboids are lengthened and inactive;
Posterior deltoid is lengthened.

Lifestyle factors that may contribute to kyphotic posture

Lack of confidence and self esteem;
Looking down at the floor when walking;
Working in an office and spending long, continual periods of time working at a desk and using a keyboard;
Working as a driver and spending long periods of time at the wheel of a lorry or car;
Having large breasts (women). Teenage girls developing breasts earlier than classmates may round shoulders to hide their development;
Being tall. Teenagers who are taller than other classmates may round over to disguise their height;
Pushing a pram or buggy;
Carrying a baby in the arms and breast-feeding;

Being very tall;

Low bone density/osteoporosis.

Kyphosis can dramatically decrease the effectiveness of transmission of the body weight down through the lower spine and limbs. It can also decrease stability and balance (contributing to falls in older adults).

Recommendations to manage and improve kyphotic posture

Align the neck;

Increase mobility of the thoracic spine and ribcage;

Strengthen the lower and middle trapezius, rhomboids and posterior deltoid muscles;

Lengthen and stretch the upper trapezius;

Develop flexibility in the pectorals and anterior deltoid;

Balance strength and flexibility of the muscles around the shoulder girdle;

Strengthen core stabilisers of pelvic and shoulder girdle;

Promote neutral pelvic alignment;

Promote thoracic breathing to assist with development of mobility.

Movements to limit kyphotic posture

Flexion of the thoracic spine. However, the first part of a half roll down (Keane, 2005) could be used (initially using the wall for support). This will develop body awareness and emphasise the restacking of the spine, engagement of lower trapezius and alignment of the neck during the return to the start position;

Lengthening of the middle trapezius, rhomboids, posterior deltoid;

Strengthening exercises for pectorals and anterior deltoid.

Note: People with kyphosis will probably experience difficulty with lateral breathing due to immobility of the spine.

Recommended exercises

- Seated spine twists (4.1) and standing
- All fours cat peddle (6.8)
- Prone lying leg raise (5.8)
- Gluteal bracing (5.9)
- Hands and knees leg extension (5.5)
- Shoulder bridge (4.3)
- Modified standing roll down (4.4) – emphasise extension
- Prone lying dart (6.11)
- Prone lying breaststroke swim (6.12)

Scoliosis

Scoliosis occurs when there is a lateral twisting of the spine, creating either a C or S curve. It is most commonly caused by genetic factors, for example unequal leg length. However, scoliosis can also be caused by the imbalance and inactivity of muscles on one side of the body (standing with weight on one leg and/or carrying bags on one shoulder). Interventions to correct the muscle imbalance and manage scoliosis should be prescribed by a physiotherapist as it will present differently between individuals.

Sway back posture

Fig. 7.6	Sway back posture

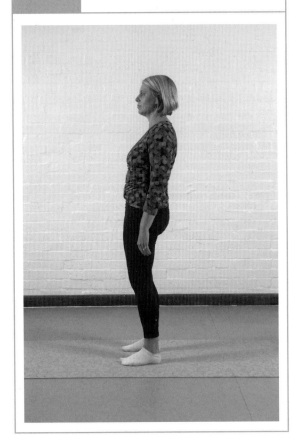

In this posture type, the hip joint is pushed forwards of the desired plumb line position (lengthening the hip flexor), but the anterior superior iliac spine (ASIS) and posterior superior iliac spine (PSIS) are level or horizontal. A hollowing or extension of the spine occurs higher up in the thoracic region of the spine. Sway back posture gives the appearance of the hips being pushed forwards and the upper back leaning backwards.

Summary of observable features of sway back posture

Head and chin poking forwards from plumb line;
  Weak neck flexor muscles;
  Cervical spine is slightly flexed;
  Thoracic spine is slightly flexed (kyphotic);
  Thoracic spine is swayed back from plumb line;
  Weakened or lengthened thoracic spine extensors;
  Lumbar spine is flexed and flattened;
  Pelvis is forward of plumb line. May be tilted backwards (PSIS may be lower than ASIS), but could also be neutral;
  Hip flexors are weaker and lengthened;
  Gluteals are shortened and weakened and may be loose or wobbly (without tone);
  Superficial abdominals may be short and tight in upper regions but weak in lower regions;
  Tensor fascia latae may be shortened;
  Knee joint can be hyperextended/locked backwards;
  Hamstring muscles can be shortened and strong.

Lifestyle factors that may contribute to sway back posture

Standing for long periods of time with the weight on one leg;
  Sometimes referred to as teenage posture.

Recommendations to manage and improve sway back posture

Stand correctly with neutral pelvis, lengthening the spine, with weight equally distributed between feet;
  Promote upright posture;

Strengthen the muscles that flex the neck;
Strengthen trapezius;
Mobilise the thoracic spine;
Mobilise the lumbar spine;
Stretch and lengthen the hamstrings and gluteals;
Strengthen the erector spinae;
Stretch the pectorals and anterior deltoid.

Recommended exercises

- Focus on standing correctly (chapter 1);
- Heel raises from standing;
- Single leg balance (standing raise) – focus on less dominant side;
- Arm float variations (6.1-6.6);
- Prone lying dart (6.11);
- Prone lying breaststroke swim (6.12)
- Shoulder bridge (4.3);
- Hip flexor stretch (5.16/5.17);
- Hamstring stretch (5.12/5.15);
- Child pose/shell stretch (4.10)
- Cat stretch (4.12)
- Supine lower back release (4.11)
- Curl-up (4.7)

Fig. 7.7   Winged scapulae

Winged scapulae

The scapulae traditionally lie flat against the ribcage and are of equal distance from the thoracic spine. A winged scapula occurs when the inner (medial) edge and lower tip stick out and away from the ribcage. This may be caused by an injury or it may be due to muscle imbalance and weakness resulting in poor posture, such as rounding the shoulders forwards and hunching the spine.

Features of winged scapulae:

Weak lower and middle trapezius and rhomboids;
Weak or inactive serratus anterior;
Tightening of the pectoralis minor, levator scapulae and rotator cuff muscles.

Recommendations to manage and improve a winged scapula

Strengthen the middle trapezius and rhomboids (dart);
Lengthen and stretch the pectoralis minor;
Strengthen the lower trapezius (dart);
Strengthen and activate the serratus anterior to help keep the scapula flat on the ribcage (Hately-Aldous, 2005:23).

Recommended exercises

- Arm float variations (6.1-6.6);
- Prone lying dart (6.11);
- Prone lying breaststroke swim (6.12);
- Shoulder bridge (4.3);
- All fours cat peddle (6.8);
- Supine lying chest stretch (6.10).

Bow legs and knock knees

Fig. 7.8	Knock knees

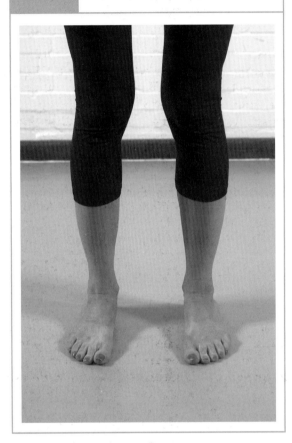

Flat feet

Flat feet (pes planus) are present when the arches of the feet are collapsed. Flat feet are apparent when walking on sand, when the whole foot shape is visible.

Flat feet can be corrected by picking up small objects (such as coins) from the floor with the toes.

Fig. 7.9	Flat foot

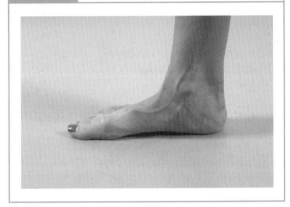

Fig. 7.10	High arch

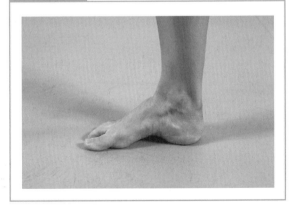

Bow legs (genu varum) describes a posture in which there is a space between the knees when the medial/inner ankle bones (malleoili) touch.

In knock knees (genu valgrum), there is a space between the inner/medial ankle bones (malleoli) when the knees are together.

Corrective exercise for bow legs and knock knees should be provided by a physiotherapist.

Assessments for muscle imbalance

Table 7.4	Assessments for muscle imbalance
Assessment for	**Assessment procedures**
Lengthened gluteus maximus 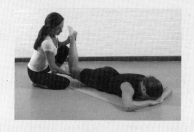	1. Lie prone, with one knee bent to a 90 degree angle. 2. Instructor raises the client's knee from floor by cupping their hand around the knee. The other hand can be placed on the pelvis lightly to check if any movement occurs (the spine should not be hyperextended). 3. Instructor counts 1, 2, 3 and releases their hand from beneath the knee on 3. (*Note:* The client should be informed of this process.) 4. The individual should be able to hold the leg in place for about 10 seconds without dropping it. The contraction of the gluteus maximus will be visible.
Shortened hip flexor/ rectus femoris 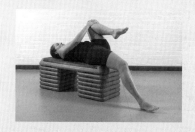	1. Lie on the edge of a table and flex one hip so the knee is raised towards the chest (the knee is also flexed). 2. The other leg hangs naturally from the edge of the table. If the extended thigh maintains a horizontal position, this usually indicates that there is no shortening of either muscle. If the thigh lifts upwards slightly (flexes), this implies that there is shortening of either the hip flexor or rectus femoris. Straightening the knee of the hanging leg can indicate which muscle is shortened: • Rectus femoris is shortened if, when the knee is straightened, the leg lowers to a horizontal position. • Iliopsoas is shortened if, when the knee is straightened, the leg does not drop and remains in a slightly raised position.

Table 7.4	Assessments for muscle imbalance (cont.)
Assessment for	**Assessment procedures**
Shortening of pectoralis minor	1. Lie supine, with the back on the floor and knees bent. 2. Place the hands at the side of the body. There should be a space between the floor and the acromion process equivalent to the width of 3 to 4 fingers. This should ideally be equal on both sides.
Shortening of pectoralis major	1. Lie supine on the back with the knees bent. 2. Place the hands at the side of the body in a 'pec dec' or 'W' position. The hands, forearm and elbow should contact the floor equally.
Lengthened lower trapezius	1. Lie prone with the tummy on the floor. 2. Position the hands at the side of the body. 3. Lift the persons shoulder blade off the floor and place in the optimal position. 4. Count to three and release the hold. The person should be able to hold the scapula in that position for approximately 10 seconds.

Adapted from Northern Fitness and Education, *Modern Pilates Stage 2* (2004)

BREATHING

8

We breathe 24 hours a day from the moment we are born till the moment we die. Breathing is the life-giving process by which we take in oxygen and remove carbon dioxide from the lungs. We breathe in (inspiration) to supply the body with oxygen, to replenish the body cells and provide a source for energy production. We breathe out (expiration) to remove carbon dioxide, a waste product of aerobic respiration.

During inspiration, the air passes through the nose and mouth to the pharynx (throat) and larynx (voice box) and down the trachea (main windpipe). It then enters the lungs (via the bronchus, which branches from the trachea – to the right and left lung into the bronchioles) and reaches the air sacs (alveoli), which are positioned at the end of the bronchioles.

Surrounding the alveoli are small blood vessels (capillaries), where 'gaseous exchange' occurs. Oxygen passes through the capillary walls into the red blood cells, to be circulated for usage around the body. Carbon dioxide is taken into the alveoli to be removed during expiration. The passage of air is reversed during expiration.

The lungs are housed and protected inside the thoracic cavity/ribcage:

At the rear of the cavity, they are protected by the thoracic spine;

At the front, they are protected by the sternum;

At the sides, they are protected by the ribs.

The diaphragm – one of the main breathing muscles – forms the lower floor that seals the thoracic cavity and is shaped like an umbrella (Coulter, 2001). When the diaphragm is relaxed, it is pressed upwards into the thorax by the abdominal contents. When it contracts, it slides down. As it does so, it either expands the abdominals (as during abdominal breathing), or doesn't expand them (as during thoracic/lateral breathing). Coulter (2001: 74-125) gives an in-depth explanation of how the diaphragm operates during different methods of breathing.

The intercostals – another of the major breathing muscles – attach between the ribs. When relaxed, they move the ribcage inwards so that the volume of the thorax and the attached lungs is at its minimum. When contracting, they move the ribcage outwards and upwards. Again Coulter (2001) offers a more in-depth explanation of these processes for those interested.

Table 8.1	
Inspiration	Expiration
Diaphragm contracts and descends	Diaphragm relaxes and ascends
Intercostals contract, moving the ribcage upwards and outwards	Intercostals relax, moving the ribcage downwards and inwards
The volume of the thoracic cavity increases and the lungs are stretched	The volume of the thoracic cavity decreases and the lungs return to their smallest size
Air pressure inside the lungs decreases	Air pressure increases in the lungs
Air enters the lungs	Air leaves the lungs

Most breathing is involuntary and unconscious. It occurs as a consequence of nerve impulses that originate from the respiratory centre of the brain and that respond to changes in the concentration of carbon dioxide (chemical stimuli). The rate of breathing for a healthy adult at rest is about 12-16 times per minute. A comparatively small volume of air is breathed in and out in one breath (tidal volume). About 0.5 litres are moved per breath or about 6 litres per minute.

During exercise, the breathing rate will increase in response to the higher demand for energy production and an increase in carbon dioxide. The contractile force of the main breathing muscles will also be greater, so the depth and speed of breathing and the volume of air moved will increase.

Some additional muscles that attach to the ribcage will also provide assistance to the respiratory muscles to move the ribcage. For forced inspiration, these include pectoralis minor and the scalenes.

For example, place the hands lightly on the collarbones. Imagine you are about to experience a sensation of being shocked or surprised (for instance, when something makes you jump) and take a breath in. You will feel the collarbones rise (see p. 141 on clavicular/thoracic breathing).

In the case of forced expiration, the additional muscles include the abdominals and the internal intercostals and subcostals.

For example, place the hands gently at the base of the ribs. Purse the lips and blow out as if blowing on a straw. You will be able to feel the abdominals working to force the breath out in this way.

Strong emotions such as fear, anger, anxiety, excitement and grief can also stimulate increased breathing rates via connections and communication between the primitive limbic system in the brain and the medulla and the bridging neurons to the hypothalamus.

We can also stimulate our breathing voluntarily and consciously using signals directly from the cerebral cortex – the thinking part of the brain. For example, we can hold our breath to duck under water or avoid an unpleasant odour. We can also take a deeper breath to enjoy the freshness and more pleasant odours during a country walk However, conscious breathing cannot be maintained for long durations because as soon as carbon dioxide levels rise the medulla initiates breathing.

Breathing and the Pilates method

The Pilates method to some extent exploits the voluntary control of breathing to fix and stabilise the muscles of the trunk during movements. The pattern of breathing recommended for most exercises in this book is to:

- Breathe in to prepare for movement;
- Breathe out and move on the effort, connecting the pelvic floor and abdominal muscles to stabilise;
- Breathe in to return back to the start position.

In most instances, the effort will be the concentric (lifting) phase of the movement. However, in some instances the effort may be on the eccentric (lowering) phase of the movement and it is recommended that participants avoid holding their breath. Care should be taken when breathing on the eccentric phase that the abdominals are engaged sufficiently so the placement of the ribcage is not compromised (for example, not poking the ribcage forwards).

O'Byrne (2006:28) suggests that during yoga and Pilates exhalation is encouraged when the spine flexes, because during the exhalation phase the ribcage closes in and the spine will naturally flex very slightly. The reverse will occur on the inhale. Spinal extension will be encouraged. Thus, the breath is used to move freely with the movement actions.

But she also suggests that this is sometimes reversed in Pilates to maintain the abdominal engagement and protect the lumbar spine. For example, during foot drops from the table top position, the movement of the foot away from the body to the floor occurs on the exhale. The moving lever (leg) can potentially create a pull on the lumbar spine (that is, cause hyperextension), so it is essential that the abdominals are engaged to prevent this. However, O'Byrne also proposes that inhaling on the extension during Pilates could be used as a challenge to the abdominals.

Methods of breathing

Clavicular/thoracic/upper chest breathing (upper)

This is where the breath is drawn into the upper chest. Latey (2001:54) refers to this as 'siphon' breathing, which she suggests 'overuses the upper accessory muscles of respiration, the scaleni, plus the trapezius, levator scapulae and serratus posterior superior posterior'.

Alternatively, Coulter (2001:102) describes two versions of this breathing: empowered thoracic breathing and constricted thoracic breathing. The former he suggests can be a useful way of inhaling as much as you can to exercise the chest during some standing yoga postures. The latter he describes as being 'typically shallow, rapid and irregular' and associated with stress and tension (2001:203).

Lateral/thoracic/diaphragmatic breathing (middle)

The method of breathing traditionally advocated for Pilates involves expanding the lower ribcage to the sides and the back during inhalation, with the abdominals still and held in static contraction. Coulter (2001:82) refers to this method as 'thoraco-diaphragmatic' breathing and he provides an explanation of how the diaphragm moves differently to accommodate this method of breathing. Latey (2001:55) describes this method of breathing as 'bellows' breathing.

This type of breathing can be felt by placing the hands lightly around the lower ribcage (thumbs at the back and hands wrapping around so that the fingers meet in front). During inspiration, the ribcage will expand laterally (to the sides) and also to the rear. During expiration, the ribs will relax.

Abdominal/diaphragmatic breathing (lower)

In this breathing method the air and diaphragm are drawn into the abdominal region and there is little movement of the ribcage. Coulter (2001:82) describes this method as 'abdomino-diaphragmatic' breathing and indicates that it is sometimes referred to as abdominal or belly breathing because this is where it can be seen and felt.

Latey (2001:55) refers to it as 'piston' breathing, which she suggests has been avoided in traditional Pilates due to the mis-interpretation that it involves 'belly-bulging' and the use of intra-abdominal pressure. In her modern Pilates method she advocates the use of both bellows and piston breathing – which she calls 'alert torso breathing' – with the engagement of muscles exaggerated on exhalation to promote their effective work.

This type of breathing can be seen and felt by placing one hand lightly on the abdominals. During inspiration, the tummy will rise lightly, not forcibly; during expiration, it will fall.

Breathing for relaxation

Abdominal or diaphragmatic breathing can be used easily and comfortably for relaxation because the muscles of the abdominals do not have to engage during relaxation. It is also probably an easier method of breathing to learn as it can be seen and felt relatively easily. However, Coulter (2001:120) suggests that, because the mind's focus is at the pelvic region, too much of this breathing pattern could induce a 'depressed, overly relaxed sensation'. Alternatively, he suggests that upper chest breathing focuses the mind upwards and creates headiness and realms of thought that are not wanted for meditation.

In one of the programmes I deliver, I begin the session with a floor-based relaxation. I teach abdominal breathing first and then teach the lateral method, with abdominals lightly engaged. Coulter suggests that, in the supine lying position, greater attention is needed to perform lateral breathing. It can therefore be useful as a 'concentration exercise' and for combining with breathing ratios.

I have also on some occasions taught upper chest breathing as a start point for breathing. My aim is to help individuals develop awareness of the different breathing methods and recognise the different effects these methods have on their physical, mental and emotional self.

Sometimes I have included the practice of a combination of each of the breathing methods during relaxation (not meditation), as a way of encouraging a fullness to the breath. An example is breathing in through the nose. Take the air down to the abdominals, expand the ribs laterally and backwards and encourage the chest to open and fill, breathing out to reverse this sequence.

Coulter (2001:120) suggests that the

preferred method for meditation is thoraco-diaphragmatic breathing (lateral breathing), because it focuses the mind centrally and can therefore balance the polarities of flighty headiness of upper chest breathing and depressive, over relaxation of abdominal breathing. *Note*: Meditation is usually performed in a seated position with the spine lengthened. This is rarely practised in Pilates classes, but is sometimes done in yoga classes.

Methods for developing breathing awareness

To raise awareness of lateral breathing

Using a band or scarf around the centre can be a useful way of raising awareness of the ribs expanding laterally. This can be performed lying, standing, seated or kneeling. Wrap the scarf around the lower ribcage. Cross the ends of the scarf in front of the body, holding them with each hand. During inhalation the scarf will become tighter, and during exhalation it will release.

To raise awareness of abdominal breathing

Place the hands on the tummy, with middle fingers touching at the belly button. During inhalation the middle fingers will separate slightly, and during exhalation they will return together.

Crook supine lying with book: Place a book across the lower abdomen. Inhale to breathe into the abdomen and expand into the pelvic floor. Exhale, drawing the abdominal area inwards and upwards. The book lowers (Latey, 2001).

To raise awareness of the difference between abdominal and lateral breathing

Spine lying with sandbag: Coulter (2001) suggests using a sandbag to raise awareness of, and strengthen, the diaphragm. He proposes using a lighter sandbag to develop abdominal breathing (3–15 pounds) and a heavy sandbag to develop diaphragmatic breathing (20–30 pounds). The heavier weight is harder to lift and encourages lateral, thoraco-diaphragmatic breathing.

Breathing ratios to assist relaxation

Yogis recommend the use of breathing ratios to assist with relaxation and move towards meditation. A ratio of 2:1 is recommended by Coulter (2001:91), whereby twice as long is taken to exhale than inhale – for example, breathing in for one count and breathing out for two counts.

This type of breathing is advocated for relaxation because it uses activities (breathing) that can be controlled consciously to affect other systems that can't. For example, slowing breathing improves the intake and delivery of oxygen, reducing the demand for the heart to work so fast (heart rate decreases). This in turn can help deal with physical and mental stress.

With this in mind, the advice is offered to keep the breathing ratios within realistic bounds so as not to cause distress, which would have an adverse effect on the heart rate! Coulter suggests an extreme would be trying to reduce the breathing to five cycles per minute (instead of the average 12–16 cycles) by using a 2:1 ratio of four-second inhale and eight-second exhale.

MIND AND EMOTIONS

9

Mental well-being

Becoming aware of the way we think is another key step towards developing self-esteem and taking care of our mental and emotional well-being.

The way we internally 'speak to' and think about ourselves, and the messages we send ourselves, will reflect how we feel and how our body appears. For example, if our thinking processes are negative and we tell ourselves we are stupid, clumsy or not good enough, this will affect how we feel, making us, say, sad, angry or disappointed. It may also be reflected in the way we carry our body (closed and hunched). Alternatively, if we think positively about ourselves – we are capable, we can handle things, we are intelligent – then we are more likely to feel happier and this again can be reflected in our bodily posture (open and upright).

The notion of having voices inside that speak to us may for some people seem a little crazy, and to some extent it may well be, depending on what and how we hear! However, the voices are there and they are fairly natural. Try the mind awareness activity below.

MIND AWARENESS ACTIVITY

Stop what you are doing, sit still and become aware of the thoughts entering your mind.

If you think to yourself 'I'm not thinking anything' or 'this is stupid' then recognise these are thoughts!

Continue to stay aware of all the thoughts that go though your mind, writing them down if necessary. Just notice how you speak to yourself without judging the processes.

Do this regularly, and start becoming aware of how you think.

Adapted from Lawrence (2005)

Thoughts pass through our minds so quickly that most of our inner talk is beyond our awareness. Those people who are aware of their thinking some of the time are more than halfway towards improving their situation. The way we think really makes a difference. It acts like a self-fulfilling prophecy: the more we see something as bad or awful, the worse it gets!

If on the other hand we can stop our thought processes before we get carried away and create a whole negative story, then we may be able to see more positives in the situation. The art of positive thinking is as many self-help writers suggest fake it until you make it! That is, think positive thoughts, even if you don't believe them at first. If you keep putting positive thoughts in, then positive thoughts come out. If you choose to put negative thoughts in, all you will see is more negatives.

Awareness of the thoughts we think and the inner workings of the mind is the key to learning to become your own best friend. At the end of the day, if we can't be our own best friend, no one else will be able to do it for us.

Fortunately, we can choose how we speak to ourselves if we are aware. Without this awareness, we can experience inner conflicts and disturbances that throw our emotions totally out of balance.

Emotional well-being

Emotions are a source of energy in motion! Safe expression is essential for our emotional well-being. Our awareness of our 'emotional' state and well-being can be outside our personal 'consciousness'. That is, we may be out of touch with what we are feeling due to suppression, denial and repression and/or other mechanisms we use consciously or unconsciously in an attempt to defend ourselves against feeling and experiencing the intensity of our emotions. Our need to hide from, or guard against, our own emotions can be due to our social and cultural background (for example, the British 'stiff upper lip') or our personal beliefs (it is not okay to express emotion). It can also stem from our inability to communicate these emotions safely and respectfully (assertiveness).

Our body, however, can reflect our emotional state. For example, when we're happy it is natural to jump for joy; when we're sad it is natural to cry. Without this expression, the emotions will be stored and can contribute to disease (stress contributes to chronic heart disease and high blood pressure, for example).

Theory to practice – application

The awareness of physical positioning encouraged by the Pilates method may draw our attention to emotional functioning and thinking. If we become more aware, attentive and nurturing towards our emotional state, and more conscious of our thinking state, we may potentially be able to free some of these tensions. We can express emotions assertively when and where we feel them – 'I feel…' – and stop any negative thinking patterns before they get a grip. This may consequently release those tensions physically as well.

Alternatively, it can operate in reverse. Working on our physical positioning and correcting our posture and alignment may help free our emotions physically. Most people who exercise regularly are aware of how much better they feel when they have finished their session. Physical movement can release emotions that have been pent up physically.

From another perspective, consciously changing our muscular positioning may affect how we feel. For example, if we concentrate on standing up straight just before a job interview our confidence may increase. Or, if you feel grumpy or sad, try looking into a mirror and smiling or laughing – it can create a shift in your emotional state.

Note: A variety of techniques for raising awareness of mental and emotional well-being are discussed in my *Complete Guide to Exercising Away Stress* (A & C Black, 2005). Some relaxation techniques from the book are described below.

Techniques for developing mental and emotional awareness

Relaxation

Providing time for relaxation somewhere in the session allows the body to be still and allows it a healthy rest. Relaxation can provide physical release for the muscles and joints and other bodily systems. It can also bring a stillness to the mind, allowing it to become less fogged, so that clarity of thinking can return.

Relaxation exercises can be performed in any position that feels comfortable. The recommended positions are supine lying, with either legs straight or knees bent, or seated (meditation posture). However, it is important for individuals to be comfortable, so alternative positions (such as seated in a chair or lying in a foetal position) can also be offered.

Prior to teaching any relaxation, it is essential that the environment is warm and any distractions (for example, mobile phones) are minimised. Blankets can be used to maintain warmth and provide comfort.

At the end of the relaxation, the group's attention should be brought steadily back to the room to enable them to wake up and focus on what they will be doing next (driving home, or performing exercises if relaxation is incorporated at the start of the session).

Relaxation techniques and scripts

The following techniques and scripts are taken from *The Complete Guide to Exercising Away Stress.*

Active muscular relaxation

Active muscular relaxation involves following instructions to actively tighten, extend or move different parts of the body and then allow them to relax and be still.

Advantages

It is a useful technique for people initially learning to relax as it is a fairly simple method to learn and can raise body awareness. This can be a particularly important skill for persons who lack body awareness and carry a lot of tension in their body posture to learn. It can help them to find active ways of releasing some of that tension. It also has the advantage that it requires little imagination.

Disadvantages

Individuals with low body awareness may find it difficult to isolate different body parts when they first use this technique. The technique is also inappropriate for persons with injuries or certain physical disabilities. A further disadvantage is that tensing the body part prior to releasing tension may actually increase tension and make it harder to relax.

Active muscular relaxation script

Sit or lie in a comfortable position.
Allow your body to relax and lengthen.
Allow your muscles to soften.
Focus your awareness on your breathing.
Notice the depth and pace of your breathing.
Allow your breathing to become slower, softer and deeper.
Take your mind's awareness to your body, starting with the feet.
Spread and separate your toes, feeling the tension in your feet.

Flex your toes towards your knees, feeling the tension in the lower leg.

Stay aware of the tension and breathe steadily in and out.

Let your toes and feet relax and let go of any tension in your lower legs.

Be still and breathe softly and deeply.

Take your mind's awareness to your thigh muscles.

Allow the muscles at the front of your thigh to tighten without locking your knee.

Tighten the muscles at the back of your thigh.

Squeeze your buttocks tight.

Stay aware of the tension in your thighs and buttocks and breathe steadily in and out.

Then let your thigh and buttock muscles relax.

Feel your hip joint open and soften.

Feel the whole of your legs relax and soften.

Be still and breathe softly and deeply.

Focus your mind's awareness on your abdomen.

Draw your abdominal muscles in tightly towards your backbone.

Feel the sides of your abdomen draw in tight.

Feel the muscles of your lower back tighten.

Stay aware of the tension and experience the feeling of a corset tightening around the centre of your body. Breathe steadily in and out.

Then release the tension in these muscles. Feel the centre of the body relax and let go.

Be still and breathe softly and deeply.

Focus your awareness on your shoulders and upper back.

Squeeze your shoulders towards the ears.

Feel the tension increase in the muscles of your upper back and the back of your neck, and breathe steadily in and out.

Allow the muscles to let go and release.

Lengthen your ears away from your shoulders.

Feel your chin tucking towards your body.

Feel the muscles in between your shoulder blades drawing downwards and tightening.

Stay aware of the tension and breathe steadily in and out.

Release the tension in these muscles and allow your body to let go.

Be still and breathe softly and deeply.

Focus your awareness on the muscles of your arms.

Extend your arms. Tense all the muscles in your upper and lower arms and breathe steadily in and out.

Clench your fists to increase the tension.

Stay aware of the tension and breathe steadily in and out.

Allow the muscles to release and let go.

Spread your fingers and open up your hands.

Extend your fingers as far away from your shoulders as you can.

Stay aware of the tension in the muscles of your hands and arms. Breathe steadily in and out.

Then release and let go and allow your arms to soften and relax.

Allow your body to be still. Breathe slowly and deeply.

Focus your mind's awareness on your face and head.

Open your mouth wide and feel the tension around your mouth and jaw.

Stay aware of the tension and breathe steadily in and out.

Then release and let go, allowing your jaw to relax. Wiggle your jaw a little.

Stick out your tongue, then allow it to relax back into your mouth.

Feel your tongue soften and your mouth and jaw relax. Breathe steadily in and out.

Wiggle your nose and then release.

Feel your eye sockets opening and then release.

Move the muscles in your forehead, then allow them to soften and relax.

Let your body sink deeper and relax further.

Let any tension just ease away.

Tighten your whole body one last time, extending your head and toes and fingers as far away from each other as you can.

Release and let go and allow yourself to sigh.

Take your mind's awareness back to your breathing.

Focus on slower, deeper breathing.

Allow your body to be still and silent.

With every breath, allow your body to relax further.

Allow a feeling of relaxation and calm to spread through your whole body.

Passive muscular relaxation

Passive muscular relaxation involves using the mind to focus on different body areas and using this awareness to relax each body part. There is no specific movement of any body part.

Advantages

Individuals who are able to focus and concentrate all their attention on their body will find this method very relaxing and calming. It is great for providing stillness to people who are very active. It is also a very effective method for people who have injuries or physical disabilities that make it uncomfortable or impossible to move specific body parts.

Disadvantages

This method may be frustrating for people who are very active and find it difficult to be still and relax. Individuals who find it difficult to focus may also struggle with the imagery of letting the specific body parts relax.

Passive muscular relaxation script

Sit or lie in a comfortable position. (See relaxation and meditation postures on p. 146.)

Allow your body to relax and lengthen.

Allow your muscles to soften.

Focus your awareness on your breathing.

Notice the depth and pace of your breathing.

Allow your breathing to become slower, softer and deeper.

Take your mind's awareness to your body, starting with your feet.

Allow your feet to soften and relax and let go of any tension.

Allow your ankle joint to open and relax.

Feel your calf muscles and the muscles at the front of your shin soften.

Take a deeper breath and, on the outward breath, allow your lower leg to relax and soften even further.

Take your mind's awareness to your knee joint.

Allow your knee joint to open and relax.

Feel the muscles at the front of your thigh soften.

Feel the muscles at the back of your thigh lengthen and relax.

Take a deeper breath and, on the outward breath, allow the whole of your legs to relax and let go.

Focus your mind's awareness on your hip joint.

Allow your hip joint to open up and relax.

Feel your buttock muscles relax and soften.

Feel the muscles around your hip release and open.

Focus your mind's awareness on your spine.

Start at the base of your spine and be mindful of each vertebra up to your skull.

Feel each vertebra open up.

Allow the muscles around your vertebrae (spine) to relax and lengthen.

Allow all the tension to ease away.

Allow your shoulder blades to separate and open up.

Take a deep breath and allow your whole spine to lengthen and relax.

Focus on your abdominal muscles.

Allow them to release.

Notice how your breath fills your abdominal area.

Observe your abdomen rising and falling with each breath.

Notice your ribcage and your breastbone.

Feel the muscles around your ribs relax.

Allow your breath to become slower and deeper.

Allow your ribs and your breastbone to soften.

Focus your awareness on your shoulder joint.

Allow your shoulder joint to open up and relax.

Feel the muscles of your upper arm lengthen and relax.

Notice your elbow joint.

Feel your elbow joint relaxing and opening.

Feel the muscles of your forearm relax and soften.

Notice your wrists and your hands.

Allow the tension to ease away.

Allow your fingers to curl open and the tension to float away.

Focus your mind's awareness on your head.

Allow each of your facial muscles to soften and relax.

Feel your jaw relax.

Feel your tongue soften.

Feel your lips gently touching and forming a soft smile.

Allow your cheek bones to relax.

Notice your eye sockets relaxing.

Allow your forehead to relax.

Allow any tension to just ease away.

Feel your body soften.

Allow your body to feel light and relaxed.

Take your mind's awareness back to your breathing.

Focus on slower, deeper breathing.

With every breath, allow your body to relax further.

Allow a feeling of peace and calm to spread through your whole body.

Note: On completion of relaxation, a silent period can be allowed for individual mindfulness/meditation.

Visualisation/guided fantasy relaxation

This involves following instructions to visualise specific images, people, events or environments that create a relaxed physiological response. It can also be used to take an individual on a specific fantasy journey by following specific instructions.

People:

If people are used in the visualisation, it is essential to guide the individual to a person who is still with them and who they love and trust and who is helpful towards them. The visualisation script can follow instructions such as:

- Notice that person.
- See what you are doing.
- Notice what you are wearing.
- Look at their face.
- Recognise any good feelings you experience being in that person's company.
- Hear their voice if they are speaking.
- Notice what they are saying or, for instance, their voice tone.

You can focus on a specific friend or a group of people you like to spend time with.

Events:

If events are visualised, it is essential to use an event with positive associations and memories. The visualisation script might be:

- Remember an event where you felt incredibly happy, positive and confident.
- Notice the sounds and the people around you.
- Notice what can you see, what can you hear, and the positive feelings you have inside.

Images:
If objects are visualised, they must be objects that the person has positive associations with, such as a photograph or teddy bear.

Environments:
If a specific environment is used for visualisation, it must be a place where the person has experienced a good feeling and feels safe. It could be a home environment, a favourite room, a country retreat, a garden, and so on.

Advantages

People who are able to visualise the pictures positively will experience the relaxation effectively. Providing specific instructions on what aspects of a visualisation to focus on can develop this mental awareness. Instructions can be to identify: pictures (such as the colour of leaves and flowers); sounds (perhaps the noise of treess rustling, the wind blowing, birds singing); smells (for example, of flowers, grass, the air); and sensations (such as the heat of the sun or the coolness of the wind). The instructions can touch all the body senses within the visualisation/fantasy.

Disadvantages

Some people may have a negative physiological response to certain images. For example, a sunny beach and the sea can bring a positive response for one person and a negative response for another, depending on their experience and the images their mind conjures. Visualising people can bring up distressing memories if the person is no longer present in the individual's life.

The visual images an individual conjures will very much be determined by their state of mind and experience and some care should be taken when using this method. This technique also takes time and can also evoke deeper feelings in some individuals.

Some people may not enjoy the experience of having to using their imagination.

Visualisation/guided fantasy relaxation script

Sit or lie in a comfortable position. (See relaxation and meditation postures on p. 146.)
Allow your body to relax and lengthen.
Allow your muscles to soften.
Focus your awareness on your breathing.
Notice the depth and pace of your breathing.
Allow your breathing to become slower, softer and deeper.
Take your mind's awareness to your body, starting with your feet and moving slowly upwards through your body.
If you feel any tension, just notice it and, on the outward breath, send the message for that body part to relax.
Let your body relax deeply and sink into the floor.
Notice in your mind's eye a gate.
Notice the height of the gate. What is it made from?
Walk slowly in your mind's eye towards the gate.
Beyond the gate is a beautiful garden where you feel totally safe and secure.
As you reach the gate, you see a lock and key. Notice the lock and key. What does it look like? How does it feel?
Allow your mind's eye to let you unlock and open the gate.
As the gate opens you notice the beautiful garden.
Notice the flowers you see, their colours and their smells.
Notice the gentle sounds you hear around you, such as birds singing or the wind blowing softly.
Notice the blue sky and the comfortable warmth of the sun.
Feel the warmth of the sun against your skin.

Close the gate behind you and then return your mind's focus back to the garden.

As you look into the garden you notice a tree.

Notice the type of tree you see, the size of the tree, the colours of the leaves and the trunk.

Notice the grass and flowers around the tree.

In your mind's eye allow yourself to walk towards the tree.

Notice the sounds of the grass rustling under your feet as you walk slowly towards the tree.

When you reach the tree, let yourself sit down and rest peacefully, taking in the beauty of the garden and the peaceful surroundings through all your senses.

Allow yourself five minutes to sit still and appreciate the garden and be at peace with yourself. (Note: If you are reading this script, allow participants to have silent time here. Tell them you will be silent and not speak for five minutes. On completion of the five minutes, continue the script.)

Now let yourself become aware of the sound of my voice again.

Take one last look around you and, in your mind's eye, look at the gate through which you entered the garden.

Allow yourself to get up slowly in your mind's eye and walk steadily towards the gate.

Notice the calm feelings you have from spending time in the garden.

As you reach the gate, look around once more and notice the safety of the garden.

Know that this is a place you can return to if you feel the need to retreat.

Open the gate and walk though and then lock the gate after you.

Walk away from the gate and prepare to bring your focus back into the room. Focus back on your breathing and awareness of your body.

Note: Complete an ending of the relaxation exercise here (see exercise 5.5b on p. 84).

Benson method of relaxation:

This is a great method that can be used by individuals on their own and in their own time. It was developed by Herbert Benson for people with high blood pressure. He initially suggested that individuals sit still and quietly, focus on saying the word 'one' out loud on their outward breath for a short time and just let the mind and body slow down with no specific effort.

The technique can be adapted in the following ways:
- The word 'one' can be replaced by other words that an individual may find more natural, such as: 'calm', 'peace', 'love', 'still', 'silent', 'relax', 'ohm' and so on. The word or mantra can be spoken silently within, rather than out loud. The technique can be used in everyday activities, for example when queuing at a supermarket, on the train, while out walking, at an office desk. The technique can be used while sitting, standing or lying and can easily be combined with other techniques.

Advantages

The greatest advantage is that the technique is very simple and is particularly beneficial for people who find it difficult to stop for long periods of time and just relax.

Disadvantages

This method may make some people feel a little self-conscious. Having to say a word or mantra out loud can be embarrassing. The alternative of saying the word or mantra inside without vocalising it will usually ease any embarrassment.

Adapted version of Benson method relaxation script

Sit quietly with an open body posture.

Focus on your breathing.

As you breath out, focus on a desired word ('calm', 'one', 'peace', 'relax', 'joy').

The word can be spoken out loud or quietly within.

Practice this for about 5–10 minutes, just allowing the body to relax.

At the end of this technique it is worth noting how the experience felt. A note pad can be used to jot down thoughts and feelings that arose.

SESSION STRUCTURE AND DESIGN

In this part of the book guidelines are offered for session structure. Some basic planning and health and safety considerations are stated and teaching qualities and skills summarised. These considerations are covered comparatively briefly as persons holding related exercise and fitness qualifications at level 2 should have prior knowledge of these.

SESSION STRUCTURE

10

Like all sessions, there should be a beginning, a middle section and an ending. The beginning section of a Pilates session will be referred to as the *preparatory phase*; the middle section will be referred to as the *main workout phase*; and the ending will be referred to as the *closing phase*.

The preparatory phase

This is the start of the session, where the teacher can set the scene for the main session and gauge the level and ability of the participants. During this phase it is essential that the main ABC principles are instructed to:

- Focus *awareness* of body and mind (it is acceptable to include a relaxation at the beginning of the session to assist with developing awareness);
- Establish correct *alignment* positioning and posture (see chapter 1 on starting postures and neutral pelvic alignment);
- Develop *breathing*;
- Engage the *core-centre*.

In addition, some mobility exercises can be included to promote better movement of the joints (synovial fluid), release some of the muscle tension around the joints and assist warming.

This phase can be performed from a standing position, an approach introduced by Cherry Baker in her Modern Pilates. It can also be performed from a lying position. Both are appropriate. In the latter, a relaxation component can be included. In the former, other techniques that promote a relaxed feel can be used (including some breath work and some mobility movements). The key is to ensure the main aims are achieved. That is:

- Align the body (from feet to head – see starting postures in chapter 1);
- Develop breathing;
- Engage the core;
- Focus awareness (either through a specific relaxation or by focusing the mind's concentration on specific movements – swaying on the feet, concentration on the breath and so on);
- Mobilise joints, release tension and assist warming and circulation.

Example mobility exercises (standing)

Note: The order of the exercises is not specified but you should aim for it to flow.

Table 10.1	Mobility exercises (standing)
Introduction	Standing posture and ABC
Shoulder girdle	Shoulder lift and lower (single side, alternating sides, both together). Emphasise the downward phase of the movement – for example: lifting for one count and lowering for three or lifting for two counts and lowering for four. Dumb waiter arms, retracting scapulae. The elbows are positioned at the side of the body and the arms raised in front as if holding a plate in each hand, palms up. The thumbs lead the movement of drawing the hands back, so they are out to the side of the body, level with the waist. Shoulder circles backwards and forwards, with the emphasis on the backwards movement.
Shoulder joint	Arm floats to front (shoulder height) Arm floats to side (shoulder height) Arm floats over head – front and side
Neck	Chin pokes/slides Nose circles Rotations – right and left Half circles – front only Chin to chest and back to upright
Spine	Side bends Trunk rotations Roll downs (partial range of motion)
Lumbar spine	Pelvic tilts – forward and back Pelvic tilts – side to side
Hips and knees	Knee raises/squats
Ankles and feet	Heel raises Shifting the weight forwards (big toe and little toe) and backwards (heel) Shorting weight from right and left Foot peddles

Note: During each exercise the ABC principles should be reinforced.

Example mobility exercises (supine lying)

Note: The order of exercises is not specified but you should aim for it to flow

Table 10.2	Mobility exercises (supine lying)
Introduction	Relaxation and ABC principles
Shoulder girdle	Shoulder shrugs (see chapter 6)
Shoulder joint	Lying arm floats to front (shoulder height) Lateral arm floats to side (shoulder height)
Neck	Chin tilts Nose circles (imagine drawing a circle on the ceiling with your nose) Rotations – right and left Half circles – front only
Spine	Supine hip rolls (4.6)
Lumbar spine	Pelvic tilts (4.2)
Hips and knees	Knee raises (5.3)
Ankles and feet	Heel raises (5.2)

Note: During each exercise the ABC principles should be reinforced.

The main workout phase

This is the middle of the session. During this section it is advisable to provide a balanced programme (whole body approach). However, when working on a one-to-one basis, or with groups with specific problems, the emphasis could be placed on including the most appropriate exercises for their needs.

Ideally, the session should use exercises that encourage work from all the starting posture positions listed in chapter 1. However, once again, if working with a group with specific needs or if insufficient equipment is available to assist performance of exercises in some positions (for example, no blocks to assist those who cannot sit upright without such support), then it is acceptable to adapt the main section.

In addition, some of the start postures (side lying, kneeling, hands and knees) may be too difficult or unbalanced for some individuals and groups. In these instances it is acceptable to work from starting positions that they find easier to perform, such as supine crook lying.

However, there are also individuals and groups who do not like to, or cannot, get up and down from the floor easily. This may include some frailer older adults and/or obese individuals. In these instances it would be acceptable to adapt the programme and primarily use seated postures (with plenty of rest phases) and seated postures using a chair.

The key things to consider during the main workout phase are:

- Planning transitions so that each exercise flows smoothly from one to the other;
- Balancing the programme to include:
  a variety of start positions;
  a variety of muscle work;
  a combination of both mobility and stability (limb loaded) exercises;
  a balanced level of flexion, extension, lateral and rotation movements for the spine;
- Incorporating stretches throughout the main session – ensuring transitions are smooth and that muscles are stretched when they have finished working. This can be left for the closing phase;
- Layering information about the exercises (easy to hard) to promote inclusion of different abilities.

The closing phase

This is the end of the session. During this phase the ABC principles can be reinforced during a combination of maintenance stretches (to return the muscles worked to normal length) and developmental stretches (to improve flexibility). There can also be a relaxation and/or meditation section to further develop awareness.

By the end of this phase the participants should be returned to the feet via a series of simple and easy transitions. For example, from back lying, roll to one side, raise the knees towards the chest, press the body over to hands and knees, walk the hands back to the thighs and into a kneeling position, lunge one leg forwards and press through the front leg to come to standing. Standing posture can then be re-educated to leave the session and some further gentle mobility exercises included if desired.

At this point in the session I usually give out some tips or homework that the participants can take forwards into their daily life. Some of the suggestions I offer (not all at once) include: standing correctly when in queues; walking correctly with the head lifted and not looking down to prevent kyphosis; taking breaks when working at a desk to re-align the body and sit correctly; carrying shopping in both arms and trying to balance the weight of each bag; lifting correctly; getting into and out of a car – the possibilities here are endless!

Table 10.3	Summary of content for each phase	
Preparatory phase	**Main phase**	**Closing phase**
Relaxation/focusing	Transitions flow	Maintenance and developmental stretch
Align the body	Muscle balance	Relaxation
Develop breathing	Variety of start positions	Reinforce ABC principles
Engage the core	Mobility and stability	Homework and provide opportunities for practice in daily life (functional application)
Focus awareness	Flexibility	
Mobilise joints, release tension and assist warming/circulation	Balanced joint and spine movement	
Basic exercises	Layer information	
Can be lying or standing		

PLANNING AND TEACHING

11

Planning and preparation

The session should be planned in advance and should take into consideration the needs of individuals and the group, the environment and the equipment needed.

Individuals/group considerations

Screening

Traditional methods of screening should occur prior to persons taking part in exercise. Persons with specific medical conditions should be referred to their GP for medical clearance.

Posture assessment

A personal interview with the client to assess their posture type and also gather information that may influence posture (for example, lifestyle and stress levels) is advisable. Posture and posture types are discussed in chapter 7.

Clothing and footwear

Footwear is not needed in a Pilates session as there is no impact work. Socks can be worn to assist performance of some exercises (leg slides) However, it is better to remove these during other exercises when it is not a requirement for the legs to slide! In addition, performing the exercise with bare feet enables greater connection and awareness of the alignment, positioning and felt experience of the feet.

All clothing should be appropriately fitted, but not so tight that it restricts movement and ideally not so baggy that joint alignment is not visible (for both teacher and students). To state the obvious, any bulky jewellery should be removed prior to the session.

Environmental considerations

Floor surface

Clean, dry and free from obstructions.

Space/class numbers

It is recommended that classes are limited to a maximum of 12 participants, thus the size and shape of the room should accommodate this number. For some community programmes, leisure centres and private clubs, there is demand for the teacher to accommodate larger class numbers. In an ideal world, the teacher should be able to assert that smaller numbers enable increased care and support for individuals. A compromise for the teacher, if demanded to teach larger numbers of people, would be to keep the programme as simple as possible to prevent any unsafe and/or ineffective technique.

Mirrors

Mirrors can be useful to allow individuals to observe their own performance and can assist self-correction. However, it is wise not to become over-dependent on them and instead develop a felt sense for the movement. In addition, mirrors can only reflect the person's technique from a front view; they cannot see the rear view (position of scapulae and so on).

From a teaching perspective, mirrors are useful for the teacher so they can maintain some visual contact with other group members while they move around the room to assist individuals. The biggest disadvantage of using mirrors is that some teachers will overuse it as a teaching aid (facing the mirror for too long). It is essential that a variety of teaching positions are used to observe individuals from different angles.

Temperature

The comparatively static nature of the exercises and techniques recommended in this book demands a warmer working environment. It would not be considered safe to stretch muscles in a cold environment. Likewise, if the room is too cold it will be harder to relax and focus awareness.

Equipment considerations

Equipment

There are numerous pieces of small equipment that can be used within the session to help individuals achieve correct positioning. These include: mats, headrests, blocks, circles, stability balls, arcs, barrels, bands and light dumbbells.

All equipment should be stored and stacked safely after use. The manufacturers guidelines should be referred to when using equipment.

Lifting and moving equipment

When moving equipment, the correct lifting technique should be used.

A lifting exercise (adapted deadlift)

Purpose
- Correct lifting
- Trunk, pelvic and scapular stability
- Ribcage placement
- Hip and knee mobility
- Strengthen gluteals, hamstrings and quadriceps

Start position

Standing, with feet a little wider than hips-width apart

Instructions and teaching points

1. Inhale to prepare.
2. Exhale, engage abdominals and slide scapulae towards buttocks.
3. Keeping the, ribcage aligned, with a space between ribs and hips, bend slightly forwards at hip and then bend at knees, lowering buttocks down as if sitting towards a chair.
4. Inhale at bottom and maintain position.
5. Exhale, engage and lift up.
6. Maintain connection between ribs and hips and keep pelvis neutral.

Variations

- Isolate and perform hip bend first, then combine with knee bend (*Note:* Hip bend alone is *not* appropriate lifting technique!).
- Combine with arm float variations described in chapter 6.
- Can be used as a preparatory exercise if standing.
- Can be used as a final closing exercise.

Music

Some sessions have calming music playing in the background to create a relaxed environment. Appropriate licences should be obtained to play music.

Teaching qualities and skills

A Pilates teacher should:

- be friendly
- be approachable
- be patient
- be motivating and encouraging
- be adaptable
- have a clear speaking voice
- show the ability and willingness to listen
- have a sense of humor
- show sensitivity and ability to respond to individual needs
- have a subject knowledge
- be aware of own body, mind and self
- be able to create a relaxed and focused environment
- deliver verbal instructions in a clear and concise manner
- be a reflective practitioner.

Communication

It is essential that the teacher is able to communicate key information to the group. Individuals will need to know:

- what they should be doing (instructions, start position, ABC principles)
- when to begin the exercise (cueing)
- how they should be doing it (teaching and alignment points)
- how to adapt the exercise to meet their needs (alternatives).

There are two ways of communicating this information:

- *visually* – via demonstrations, body language, gestures, facial expressions and eye contact;
- *verbally* – via spoken instructions.

The combined usage of both visual and verbal communication strategies is usually the most effective as people learn in different ways.

It is recommended that teachers use a layered approach for providing information for each exercise and that they work with the ABC principles listed in chapter one:

- *alignment* – establishing a solid start posture and pelvic placement;
- *awareness* – promoting this throughout;
- *breathing* – establishing the breath pattern;
- *centring* – engaging the core;
- *differentiation* – offering alternatives;
- *exercise and endurance* – delivering the exercise and encouraging individuals to work at a repetition range that suits them. Individuals progressing to more advanced positions for the first time may need to be encouraged to perform fewer repetitions initially and to build this up steadily over the forthcoming weeks.

Demonstrations

A demonstration provides a visual picture of how the exercise should be performed. Demonstrations should be given in a position where all participants are able to see and be seen. It is advisable that participants are encouraged to sit correctly to observe demonstrations.

When giving a demonstration, it is essential that the teacher's body alignment and exercise technique are precise and accurate. A poor demonstration will be ineffective, since participants will have to interpret the exercise in their own way and may perform unsafely or ineffectively.

During the demonstration, the teacher should perform a couple of silent repetitions so that the group can focus just on the movement. The teacher should also offer some spoken information to emphasise key alignment and teaching points. In addition to this, the teacher may point to specific areas on their body as they move in order to draw the group's attention to a specific area.

It may not always be necessary to demonstrate every exercise, especially in classes where individual participants have more experience and skill. In these instances the teacher can use verbal instructions to talk the group into positions, through the exercise and out of positions.

Teaching position

The golden rule here is to be in a position where you can see, and be seen by, all participants at all times. It is recommended that the teacher circulates around the session and observes from different angles to identify and make corrections. When making individual corrections, the teacher should maintain contact with the rest of the class and continue to keep an eye on their practice.

Corrections

Initially the reinforcement of some key teaching and coaching points may suffice, along with eye contact and visually pointing to the teacher's own alignment to reinforce correct performance – for example, pointing to the shoulders and pressing them down to encourage this in participants.

Hands-on correction tends to be advocated and used within the Pilates method to assist performance. For example, placing the hands on an individual's shoulder blades as they perform shoulder lifts or arm floats from a standing position can help them to develop an awareness of how their body is moving.

However, hands-on correction must be undertaken with sensitivity and respect for the individuals. Some individuals are uncomfortable with being touched and thus it is wise for the teacher to state at the beginning of the class that they will be using this approach. They should also offer the opportunity for individuals to request not to be touched if they are uncomfortable. In addition, touching should never be used to jerk or pull a person's body around, or push them into positions they are not able to achieve. It is more a way of raising awareness of their alignment and assisting with development of their own felt movement sense.

As with other forms of exercise, sometimes more than one participant will need to be corrected. In these instances, the teacher should prioritise corrections to individuals performing less safely and effectively. However, it may also be wise for the instructor to review and revise how they set up the exercise and reconsider whether they layered the information and key principles sufficiently prior to the exercise being performed. Another consideration could be whether the participants were able to hear the teacher and see their demonstrations clearly. These are points the teacher can use to guide reflection on their practice.

Closing the session and evaluation

At the end of the session, the teacher should thank participants and invite questions. It is also advisable to gather information from class participants by asking open questions regarding how they experienced the session and any aspects they were unclear of. This will enable the teacher to respond to feedback by making adaptations as necessary to future sessions. By doing this, the teacher demonstrates to the class that he or she is responsive to their needs.

The teacher can also appraise and evaluate their own teaching by reviewing the session and considering which aspects they delivered clearly and which aspects could have been delivered more effectively. For example, could they be seen and heard by all participants? Were they able to offer alternatives and respond to individual needs? Evaluating one's performance is a very difficult skill. However, it is essential for developing practice and planning for future continued professional development (CPD).

EXERCISE ANALYSIS AND REVIEW OF THE ORIGINAL 34 EXERCISES 12

The key thing to remember throughout this chapter is that *not all exercises are okay for all people!*

Joseph Pilates was indeed ahead of his time in relation to developing exercise and activity. However, he worked primarily with dancers and indeed many elite performers, who would have had incredible flexibility and strength and would have been able to get into most positions without compromising their alignment too much. In addition to this, activity and health levels among the general population during the 1920s and up to 1960s were probably higher than the activity levels reported recently by the Department of Health (2005). In addition, the health statistics (incidence of obesity and CHD and so on) would have been significantly different during those years. Furthermore, there have been numerous developments in exercise and health science over the years and this area will continue to be studied, reviewed and updated in light of new evidence.

In this chapter some of the safety considerations applied to other exercise disciplines will be explored. The issues considered will include:

- individual factors
- the 'SEESAW' principle
- joint actions
- muscle actions
- the 'OK' exercise quadrant

These issues will be described initially. The modified exercises described throughout this book will then be aligned with similar exercises from the traditional method (either by 'position' – such as side lying or seated – or by 'purpose' for performing, for example lengthening hamstrings, trunk stability). People wishing to explore the traditional exercises further are advised to seek supervision and instruction from a reputable school, some of which are listed at the end of this book. It should be noted that many of these schools have moved away from teaching the traditional exercises, certainly for lower skill and fitness levels.

Individual factors

We human beings come in all shapes, sizes and genetic packaging. We differ in our life experiences, our cultures and social backgrounds, our priorities, our needs (physical, mental, emotional, nutritional, spiritual, material and so on) and our values. In addition, each of us will have a whole host of other factors that are unique to ourselves. These factors intertwine to make us the person we are on each level.

From an exercise perspective, the safety of certain exercises will be primarily dependent on some specific physical factors. However, these are not isolated factors and can have links to other levels of our being (mental, social, emotional and so on). Differences between individuals include:

- existing flexibility and ability to stretch/lengthen muscles
- existing mobility and range of motion at specific joints
- strength and endurance of the specific muscles
- over-activity/underactivity of specific muscles impacted by lifestyle factors or previous injury
- core stability of muscles supporting the pelvic girdle, trunk and shoulder girdle
- posture and posture types (lordotic, kyphotic and so on)
- joint and bone health (osteoporosis, bone density, arthritis)
- age, gender, lifestyle and work – sedentary or active
- medical conditions and injuries
- body type – (such as ectomorph). Body weight (underweight, overweight, obese), height, and length of levers are all related to body type
- storage of fat – that is, where weight is carried (apple or pear body shape)
- fitness and skill level, specificity of current training, existing activity levels, experience with the Pilates method

- individual goals, for example health-related or performance-related (athletic/dance).

Teachers should consider all of these factors before developing a programme of exercises for an individual. Once the potential level, ability and needs have been assessed, the specific exercises that may be appropriate can be reviewed using the 'SEESAW' principle. This will provide a basis for analysing the potential safety and effectiveness of the exercises.

In chapter 1, some very basic and general descriptions are offered to create levels for individuals. However, all of the aforementioned factors also need to be considered.

Note: It should be noted that, while some of the exercises described previously may seem appropriate and even 'easy' for some people, they will *not* be appropriate for everyone.

The SEESAW principles

Table 12.1	SEESAW principles

Speed

How fast is the exercise being performed?
Is the individual moving too quickly and exceeding or reaching the end of their range of motion too rapidly?
Does the exercise enable them to perform with control, or are they rushing to compete and trying to complete an exercise they are not ready for?

Equipment and environment

Does the individual need assistance with balance, for example by holding a wall? Do they need help to achieve or extend the range of motion for stretches, for example by using a strap to reduce range during a hamstring stretch?
Is the environment warm enough for stretching and relaxation exercises (cold muscles will not stretch effectively and are potentially at risk of injury)? *Note:* Layered clothing can be worn to maintain temperature and blankets can be used for relaxation.
Is the floor clean and dry? Do the mats have sufficient cushioning? Is there sufficient equipment for everyone?

Effectiveness

Is the position achieving the intended outcome, for example stretching the desired muscle? Is it mobilising the desired joint? Is it strengthening, or providing endurance for, the desired muscle? Is it challenging core stability?
Is there another exercise or range of exercises that may be more appropriate for the individual's needs, such as their postural type and level of ability? (See the discussion on differentiation in chapter 1.)

Stability

How secure is the position? This varies according to the base of support (for example, side lying is less stable than supine lying). How balanced is the individual in the position?
Are the joints in stable positions? (For example, in deep knee bending movements with the knee fully flexed, the knee ligaments are stretched and thus the joint is less stable.)

Table 12.1	SEESAW principles (contd)

Alignment

Is the body positioned correctly? Is the individual able to position their body correctly for the specific exercise? Do they sufficient strength and flexibility? Are the joints moving in appropriate anatomical direction and through correct alignment?

Does the individual have sufficient core strength to hold a position (such as a full press-up position) and maintain the integrity of the muscles around the shoulder and pelvic girdles?

Weight

How much weight or resistance is there? Individuals who are obese are already carrying additional weight. Individuals with larger legs will have greater weight in this region than those with leaner frames. This will affect their ability to perform the exercises safely and effectively.

Longer leverage and weight carried around specific levers will add resistance to movement.

When reviewing exercises using SEESAW, it is also essential to review the joints moving during the exercise in order to ensure the body is moving in a way it has been designed to.

Summary of joint actions

All exercises are limited by the directional movements that are anatomically possible at the specific joint.

Table 12.2	Mobility exercises (standing)	
Joint	**Actions**	**Example**
Knee	Flexion and extension	Bending and straightening the knee
Ankle	Plantar flexion and dorsi flexion	Pointing and flexing the foot Can also circle foot courtesy of sliding joints in ankle
Hip	Flexion and extension and hyperextension	Lift knee to hip Straighten leg Take leg behind body
	Abduction and adduction	Take leg away from midline of the body Bring leg towards the midline of the body
	Rotation	Twist hip inwards and outwards
Elbow	Flexion and extension Pronation and supination	Bend and straighten elbow Rotate palm up and down
Shoulder joint	Flexion and extension Abduction and adduction	Raise arm in front of body and back behind body Take arm away from midline of body and bring arm towards the midline of the body
	Rotation	Twist arm inwards and outwards
	Circumduction	Full arm circles
	Horizontal flexion/extension	Drawing arms towards and away from each other in horizontal plane (hugging action)
Shoulder girdle	Elevation and depression Retraction and protraction	Lift and lower shoulders Draw shoulders backwards and round them forwards
Lumbar spine	Flexion and extension	Bend and straighten back (chest moves towards pelvis)
	Hyperflexion and hyperextension	Hump and hollow

Table 12.2	Mobility exercises (standing) (contd)	
Thoracic spine	Lateral flexion and extension Rotation	Side bends Twist right and left
Cervical spine (atlas and axis)	Flexion and extension Hyperflexion and hyperextension Rotation Lateral flexion/extension	Bend and straighten (head towards chest and back to upright) Twist right and left Bend head to side and back up

Muscle actions

Another key consideration is to recognise which muscle is working and how it is working.

Here is a summary of how muscles work:

- muscles pull on bones to move the joints they cross in specific directions and according to their structure (hinge, ball and socket and so on)
- muscles work to overcome or lift resistances. Resistances include body weight, levers (arms and legs), gravity, barbells, exercise bands, pulley equipment, water and so on

- muscles contract and get shorter to lift a resistance (prime mover – concentric work)
- muscles contract and lengthen to lower a resistance (prime mover – eccentric work)
- muscles contract to hold a position (static/isometric/fixator work)
- muscles can relax to enable the opposite muscle to work (antagonist lengthening as prime mover contracts)
- muscles can lengthen and relax (active and/or passive stretching)

Note: More detailed information regarding muscle actions is provided throughout specific chapters.

Table 12.3	Summary of muscle actions	
Muscle	Joints crossed	Prime action when contracting concentrically
Gastrocnemius	Ankle Knee	Plantar flexion of ankle (pointing toe) Assist flexion of knee (bending knee)
Soleus	Ankle	Plantar flexion of ankle with knee bent.
Tibialis anterior	Ankle	Dorsi flexion of the ankle (lifting toe up towards the knee)
Hamstrings	Knee Hip	Flexion of the knee (lifting heel towards the buttocks) Extending hip (assisting gluteals)
Quadriceps	Knee Hip	Extension of the knee (straightening the knee) Flexion of hip (assisting hip flexor)
Gluteus maximus	Hip	Extension of the hip (lifting the leg behind the body)
Hip flexor	Hip	Flexion of the hip (lifting the knee to the chest)
Abductors	Hip	Abduction of the leg (taking the leg out to the side, away from the midline of the body)
Adductors	Hip	Adduction of the hip (taking the leg across the front and towards the midline of the body)
Rectus abdominis	Spine	Flexion of the spine (bending the spine forwards)
Erector spinae	Spine	Extension of the spine – (straightening the spine)
Obliques	Spine	Lateral flexion and rotation of the spine (twisting and bending the trunk to the side)
Transverses abdominis	Spine	Spine stabiliser – corset Transversus works isometrically to draw abdominal contents back towards the spine (Thompson, 1989)
Multifidus	Spine	Extension of individual vertebral section

Table 12.3	Summary of muscle actions (contd)	
Quadratus lumborum	Spine	Holds the spine in place when holding a heavy object in one hand (isometric) Lateral flexion/extension when contracting concentrically/eccentrically against resistance
Pectorals	Shoulder	Adduction of arm (drawing arm laterally across front of the body) and horizontal flexion of the arm (drawing the arms together horizontally in front of the body)
Trapezius	Shoulder girdle	Extension of neck (keeping the head up) Elevation of the shoulder (lifting shoulders to ears) Depression of scapulae (drawing scapulae downwards toward buttocks) Retraction of the scapulae (squeezing the shoulder blades together)
Latissimus dorsi	Shoulder	Adduction of the shoulder (taking the arms down laterally towards the body) Also shoulder extension, for example during chin-ups (Thompson, 1989)
Deltoids	Shoulder	Abduction of the shoulder (lifting arms out sideways) Flexion and extension of shoulder (anterior and posterior fibres)
Biceps	Elbow	Flexion of the elbow (bending the elbow)
Triceps	Elbow	Extension of the elbow (straightening the elbow)

Adapted from Lawrence, *The Complete Guide to Exercise to Music* (2004)

The OK exercise quadrant

Once the exercise has been reviewed, taking into consideration all the factors discussed previously, it can be placed into the OK quadrant. It can then be reviewed further to explore ways of modifying the exercise so that it may enter the safe and effective section.

Table 12.4	The OK exercise quadrant

Safe and effective **OK to perform** Correct exercise position, intensity and difficulty for the individual performing	**Safe and ineffective** Exercises that are too easy would be placed in this box. Ways should be sought to progress the exercise to increase effectiveness. For example, some of the exercises described as being appropriate for all levels may be easy for those of higher levels. Persons of higher levels should explore more challenging options to work effectively. Some variations and progressions are offered for specific exercises.
Unsafe and effective Check individual factors here as some exercises may be OK for some people and not OK for others. Can the exercise be modified in the following ways to raise safety and move to box 1? • Lever length • Speed • Start position • Repetitions • Resistance/gravity • Stability • Range of motion Always consider whether the risks outweigh the benefits. If they do, leave out the exercise or modify it!	**Unsafe and ineffective** Some exercises and exercise equipment are considered ineffective (that is, they do not bring about the benefits they claim). In addition, some exercises/equipment may have numerous risks attached. Exercises in this quadrant would be considered contraindicated – that is, the risk of performing them would outweigh the benefits.

The original exercise modifications

The hundred

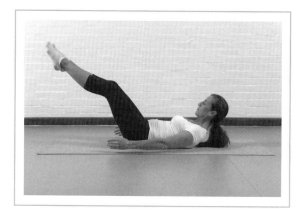

Purpose

- Abdominal endurance to maintain pelvic stability and thoracic flexion of spine

Reason for modification

If the individual has insufficient core strength, extended legs may cause hip flexor to pull on lumbar spine and create hyperextension.

Example modifications for individuals with insufficient core strength

- 4.7 Supine curl-up
- 4.8 Modified one hundred

The roll-up

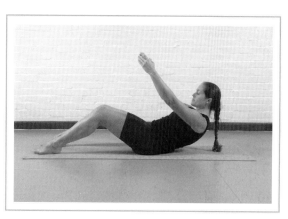

Purpose

- Spine mobility and stability
- Scapular stability
- Abdominal and hip flexor strength and hamstring flexibility

Reason for modification

If the individual has insufficient core strength, this can be adapted initially to isolate all key movements, without risking stress to lower back caused by hip flexor pull when sitting up.

Example modifications for individuals with insufficient core strength

- 4.7 Supine curl-up and build range
- 4.4 Modified standing roll down
- 5.15 Seated hamstring stretch

Rollover with legs spread

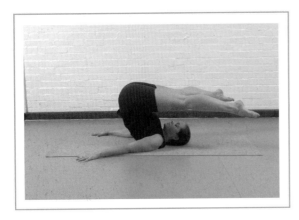

Rocking with open legs

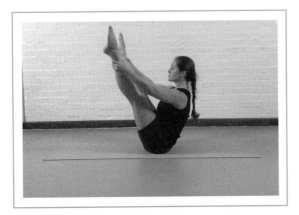

Purpose
- Mobility of spine
- Pelvic and scapular stability
- Lengthen back and hamstring muscles
- Lengthen adductors if legs spread

Reason for modification

Can be adapted to isolate all key movements, without risking stress to spine when rolling back and weight bearing (a risk for persons with low bone density in the spine). Also, shoulder girdle and cervical spine area are not designed for carrying body weight.

Example modifications for individuals with insufficient core strength
- 4.5 Modified seated roll back
- 5.15 Seated hamstring stretch
- 5.14 Seated adductor stretch
- 4.7 Supine curl-up
- 4.3 Supine lying shoulder bridge

The one leg circle

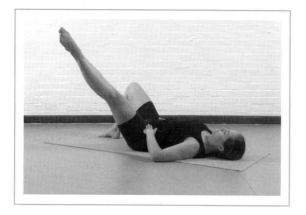

Purpose

- Hip mobility
- Stability of pelvis and spine challenged by movement of long lever

Reason for modification

Long lever with resistance of gravity can place additional stress on spine. There are easier ways to achieve hip mobility and maintain stability for persons lacking flexibility and mobility.

Example modifications for individuals with insufficient core strength

- 5.11 Supine ankle bends and foot circles to leg circle
- 5.3 Supine knee raise
- 5.4 Supine toe dips

Rolling back like a ball

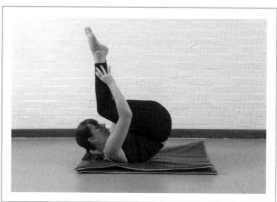

Purpose

- Maintaining stability in flexed position
- Maintaining scapular stability
- Balance in top position to sit on sitting bones

Reason for modification

Spine mobility can be achieved without weight-bearing rolling action, which would be contraindicated for persons with low bone density in the spine.

Other exercises in the series strengthen abdominals.

Example modifications for individuals with insufficient core strength

- 4.5 Modified seated roll back

Single leg stretch

Double leg stretch

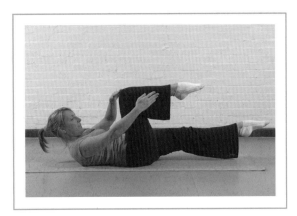

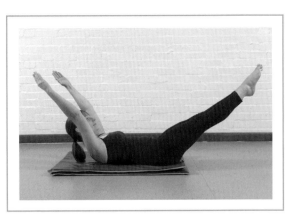

Purpose

- Hip flexor and gluteal stretch
- Hip mobility (flex and extend)
- Abdominal strength
- Co-ordination

Example modifications for individuals with insufficient core strength

Exercises listed prepare for this movement.
- 4.9 Supine single leg stretch
- 5.1 Supine crook lying heel slide
- 5.2 Supine heel raise
- 5.3 Supine knee raise/float
- 4.7 Supine curl-up
- 5.17 Supine lying hip flexor stretch

Purpose

- High levels of abdominal strength to maintain alignment with both legs extended
- Mobility of hip and shoulder
- Co-ordination

Reason for modification

Extended legs may cause hip flexor to pull on lumbar spine and create hyperextension. Arm lever may add to this.

Example modifications for individuals with insufficient core strength

- 4.9 Supine single leg stretch
- 5.1 Supine crook lying heel slide
- 5.2 Supine heel raise
- 5.3 Supine knee raise/float
- 5.17 Supine lying hip flexor stretch
- 4.7 Supine curl-up
- 4.8 Modified one hundred

The spine stretch

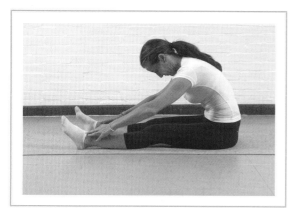

Rocking

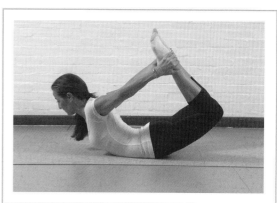

Purpose

- Stretch hamstrings and erector spinae
- Spine mobility
- Pelvic stability
- Sequential control

Reason for modification

Stretches can be isolated to achieve effective stretch of all muscles for those lacking flexibility.

Block sitting can be used for persons with tight hamstrings

Example modifications for individuals with insufficient core strength

- 5.15 Seated hamstring stretch
- 4.12 Hands and knees cat stretch (spine flexion)
- 4.11 Supine lower back release
- 4.10 Shell/child pose stretch

Purpose

- Spinal extension/mobility
- Hip flexor flexibility
- Pectoral flexibility to reach and hold ankles
- Scapular and pelvic stability

Reason for modification

Spine mobility/extension can be achieved without weight-bearing roll action (back raises). Spine is vulnerable if in hyperextension.

Example modifications for individuals with insufficient core strength

- 5.13 Quadriceps stretch (progress to double legs)
- 5.19 Prone lying leg curl
- 6.11 Prone lying dart
- 6.10 Supine lying chest stretch

Cork screw

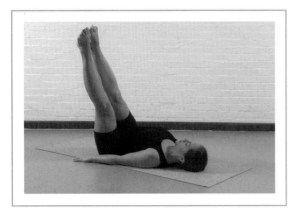

Purpose

- High levels of abdominal strength to maintain alignment with both legs extended
- Coordination (circling action)
- Spine mobility to lift and lower legs
- Pelvic and scapular stability to maintain alignment

Reason for modification

Extended legs may cause hip flexor to pull on lumbar spine and create hyperextension.

Example modifications for individuals with insufficient core strength

- 4.6 Supine hip rolls
- 5.3 Supine knee raise/float
- 5.4 Supine foot dip (table top)
- 5.11 Supine ankle bends and foot circles to single leg circle
- 4.3 Supine lying shoulder bridge

The saw

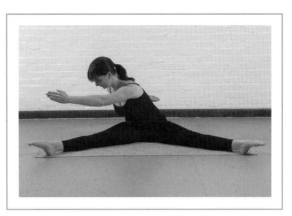

Purpose

- Spine mobility
- Hamstring and adductor flexibility
- Pelvic stability

Reason for modification

Spine mobility can be achieved in isolation and without the flexibility required by the seated straddle position.

Adductor stretch and hamstring stretch can be adapted or isolated for persons with low flexibility.

When all the above are achieved, arm leverage adds the additional focus of scapular stability.

Example modifications for individuals with insufficient core strength

- 4.1 Seated spine rotation/twist
- 5.15 Seated hamstring stretch
- 5.14 Seated adductor stretch

The swan dive

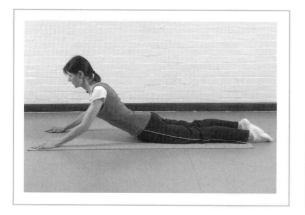

Purpose

- Spine mobility when rocking
- Gluteal and erector spinae strength and endurance to maintain position
- Shoulder girdle muscle strength to stabilise scapulae
- Chest flexibility

Reason for modification

For less skilled individuals, exercise goals can be isolated and achieved without the risk placed on the spine if moving into hyperextension with heavy limb load (arms and legs).

Example modifications for individuals with insufficient core strength

- 5.8 Prone lying leg raise (can be progressed to double leg)
- 5.9 Gluteal bracing
- 6.11 Prone lying dart
- 6.12 Prone lying breaststroke swim

Prone lying abdominal stretch with elbows resting on floor and chest lifted (not illustrated) can be progressed by extending arms fully.

One leg kick

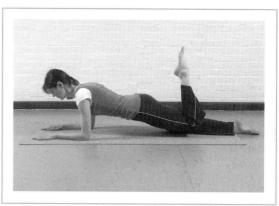

Purpose

- Pelvic stability
- Knee mobility
- Abdominal endurance to maintain neutral in lifted position
- Hamstring strength and quadriceps flexibility

Reason for modification

Can isolate leg movement and maintain spine alignment by prone lying.

Example modifications for individuals with insufficient core strength

- 5.19 Prone lying leg curl
- 5.13 Quadriceps stretch

Double leg kick

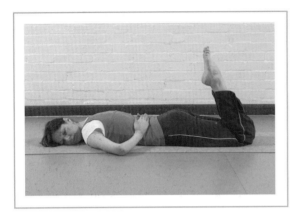

Purpose

- Hamstring strength
- Quadriceps flexibility
- Stability of pelvis and scapulae
- Strengthen erector spinae to extend spine (lifted position)

Reason for modification

Spine alignment can be maintained more easily lying prone. Perform single leg kick before progressing to double.

Example modifications for individuals with insufficient core strength

- 5.19 Prone lying leg curl
- 5.13 Quadriceps stretch

Neck pull

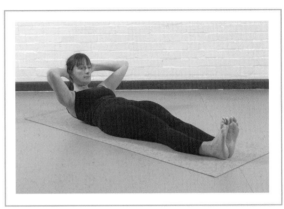

Purpose

- Abdominal and hip flexor strength
- Hamstring flexibility
- Stability of pelvis and scapulae

Reason for modification

Can be adapted to isolate all key movements, without risking stress to lower back caused by hip flexor pull when sitting up and without risking pull on neck, which would stress cervical vertebrae.

Example modifications for individuals with insufficient core strength

- 4.7 Supine curl-up
- 5.15 Seated hamstring stretch

Scissors

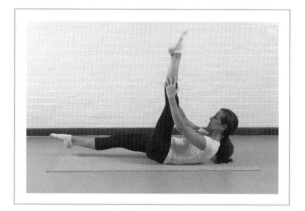

Purpose

- Hip mobility
- Abdominal strength to hold position
- Hamstring and hip flexor flexibility in lengthened position (strength/endurance when moving)

Reason for modification

Original exercise was performed in an elevated bridge position/shoulder stand position (shoulder girdle is not designed for weight bearing). Exercise goals can be achieved in isolation.

Example modifications for individuals with insufficient core strength

- 4.2 Supine pelvic tilt
- 4.3 Supine lying shoulder bridge
- 5.2 Supine heel raise
- 5.3 Supine knee raise/float
- 5.17 Supine lying hip flexor stretch
- 5.12 Lying hamstring stretch

Bicycle

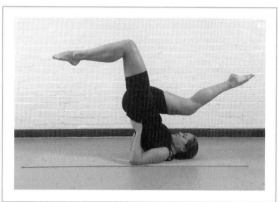

Purpose

- Hip mobility
- Pelvic and scapular stability
- Abdominal strength to hold position
- Hamstring and hip flexor flexibility
- Co-ordination

Reason for modification

Original exercise was performed in an elevated shoulder stand position (shoulder girdle is not designed for weight bearing). Exercise goals can be achieved in isolation.

Example modifications for individuals with insufficient core strength

- 5.3 Supine knee raise/float
- 4.2 Supine pelvic tilt
- 4.3 Supine lying shoulder bridge
- 5.11 Supine ankle bends and foot circles (adapt to perform cycling action with leg)
- 5.4 Supine toe dips

Shoulder bridge

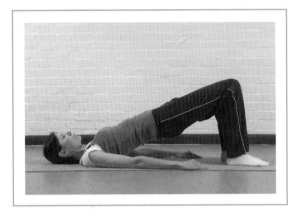

Purpose
- Spine mobility when rolling, stability when holding and weight bearing
- Sequential control and co-ordination

Reason for modification
Exercises listed progress to this exercise position.

Example modifications for individuals with insufficient core strength
- 4.2 Supine pelvic tilt
- 4.3 Supine lying shoulder bridge (with variations listed to progress)

Spine twist

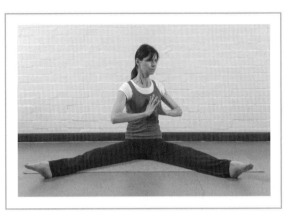

Purpose
- Spine mobility
- Hamstring flexibility to sit upright
- Pelvic and scapular stability
- Sequential control

Reason for modification
Develop flexibility to sit correctly by isolation of stretches for persons lacking flexibility. Use blocks to assist persons with tight hamstrings to sit up correctly. Legs could be crossed.
Exercises listed can progress to this.

Example modifications for individuals with insufficient core strength
- 4.1 Seated spine rotation/twist
- 5.15 Seated hamstring stretch

Jack knife

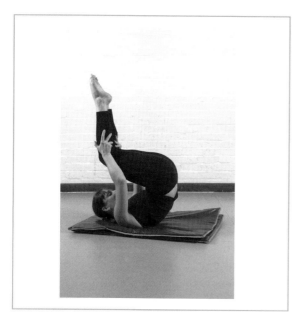

Purpose

- Spine and hip mobility
- Abdominal strength to maintain alignment and support body weight in balance position

Reason for modification

Exercise goals can be achieved in isolation without risking stress on lumbar spine. Also, shoulder girdle and cervical vertebrae bear some body weight and are not designed for this purpose.

Example modifications for individuals with insufficient core strength

- 4.2 Supine pelvic tilt
- 4.3 Supine lying shoulder bridge
- 5.15 Seated hamstring stretch
- 5.12 Lying hamstring stretch

Side leg kick kneeling

Side leg kick lying

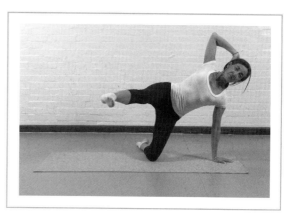

Purpose

- Hip mobility
- Ankle mobility
- Abductor strength to hold leg up
- Pelvic stability during hip movement
- Scapular stability to hold body weight if performed in side kneeling position (original)

Reason for modification

Exercise goals can be isolated. Some individuals may struggle to maintain balance and isolation necessary to perform all movements correctly.

Example modifications for individuals with insufficient core strength

- 5.2 Supine heel raise
- 5.3 Supine knee raise/float
- 5.6 Side lying outer thigh raise (can be progressed to performing resting on elbow and without dropping waist)
- 5.10 Side lying clam
- 4.14 Side plank Hold side kneeling position without leg kick.

Teaser

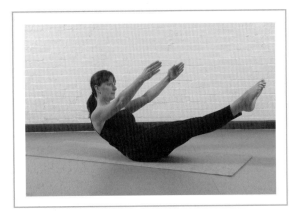

Purpose

- High level of abdominal strength
- High level of hip flexor strength to hold in top position
- Hamstring flexibility in top position
- Balance to hold top position
- Scapular stability during shoulder joint movement
- Co-ordination

Reason for modification

Exercise goals can be isolated. Risk of stress on lower back caused by hip flexor pulling lumbar spine into hyperextension on first phase.

Example modifications for individuals with insufficient core strength

- 4.7 Supine curl-up
- 4.8 Modified one hundred
- 4.9 Single leg stretch
- 5.15 Seated hamstring stretch
- 5.12 Lying hamstring stretch
- 6.1-6.6 Arm float variations

Balance in V position with knees bent (use strap to assist).

Hip twist

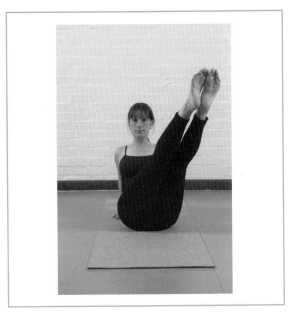

Purpose

- High level of abdominal strength
- Flexibility for chest and anterior deltoid
- Pelvic and scapular stability
- Strengthen hip flexors

Reason for modification

Exercise goals can be isolated without risking stress on lower back, which may be caused by hip flexor pulling lumbar spine into hyperextension. Hip flexor already strong.

Example modifications for individuals with insufficient core strength

- 6.10 Supine lying chest stretch
- 5.2 Supine heel raise
- 5.3 Supine knee raise/float
- 4.7 Supine curl-up
- 5.11 Supine ankle bends and hip circles (can be adapted to lifting and lowering leg)

Can be adapted and performed on elbows.

Swimming

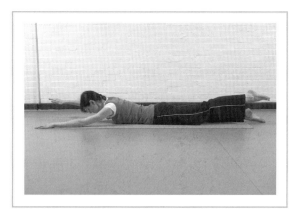

- 5.5 Hands and knees leg raise
- 6.9 Hands and knees arm reach
- 5.5 and 6.9 combined for progression

Purpose

- Hip and shoulder mobility
- Gluteal strength to extend leg
- Shoulder girdle muscle strength to extend shoulders and stabilise scapular
- Chest flexibility
- Co-ordination of movements of arms and legs

Reason for modification

Exercise goals can be isolated and achieved without risk placed on spine if moving into hyperextension with heavy limb load (arms and legs).

Example modifications for individuals with insufficient core strength

- 6.11 Prone lying dart
- 6.12 Prone lying breaststroke swim
- 5.8 Prone lying leg raise. Can be progressed to holding elevated and alternate leg raise, or adding prone lying arm raise of opposite arm, with or without arc barrel to support lumbar spine.
- 5.9 Gluteal bracing

Leg pull – prone

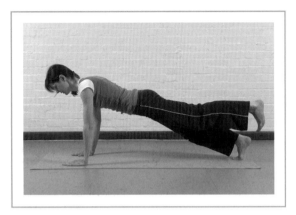

Purpose

- Upper body strength/endurance
- Scapular stability
- Abdominal strength/endurance
- Lower body strength/endurance to hold fixed position
- Gluteal strength to extend hip

Reason for modification

Exercises listed can progress to this.

Wrist extension may be uncomfortable for some individuals

Example modifications for individuals with insufficient core strength

- 5.8 Prone lying leg raise
- 5.9 Gluteal bracing
- 5.5 Hands and knees leg raise
- 6.13 Hands and knees to plank (variations listed progress intensity)
- 6.14 Hands and knees to press-up

Leg pull – supine

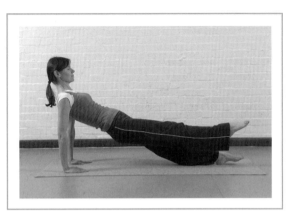

Purpose

- Upper body strength, scapular stability and chest flexibility to hold position
- Abdominal strength/endurance to maintain spine alignment
- Hip and ankle mobility
- Hip flexor strength to raise and lower moving leg

Reason for modification

Hip flexor muscles are already strong. Exercise goals can be achieved with lower limb load to reduce risk placed on spine if moving into hyperextension with heavy limb loading (long lever).

Wrist extension may be uncomfortable for some individuals.

Example modifications for individuals with insufficient core strength

- 6.10 Supine lying chest stretch
- 5.3 Supine knee raise/float
- 4.7 Supine curl-up
- 5.11 Supine ankle bends and hip circles (can be adapted to lifting and lowering leg)

From start position, lift and lower buttocks (isotonic) before moving to hold position (isometric). Start with small range of motion.

Side bend –mermaid

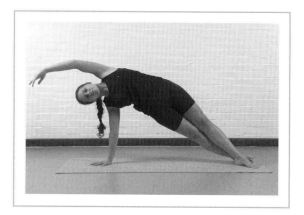

Purpose

- Upper body strength
- Abdominal strength
- Oblique stretch
- Balance – narrow base of support
- Pelvic, spine and scapular stability

Reason for modification

Exercise goals can be isolated. Some individuals may lack flexibility/strength/stability to perform correctly. Exercises listed can progress to this.

Example modifications for individuals with insufficient core strength

- 4.13 Seated side bend
- 4.14 Side plank

Boomerang

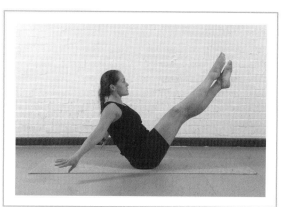

Purpose

- Shoulder mobility through horizontal flexion and extension
- Spine mobility/stability
- Hamstring and pectoral flexibility
- Co-ordination and control

Reason for modification

Mobility of shoulder girdle can be achieved without other movements. Spine mobility can be achieved without weight bearing, which is – contraindicated for persons with low bone density in the spine. Shoulder girdle is not designed for weight bearing. Stretching muscles can be isolated.

Example modifications for individuals with insufficient core strength

- 4.5 Modified seated roll back
- 5.15 Seated hamstring stretch
- 6.10 Supine lying chest stretch

Seal

Crab

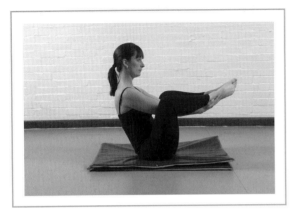

Purpose

- Stability to maintain flexion of spine
- Abdominal strength/endurance
- Balance (thoracic spine on down phase and sitting bones on lifted phase)
- Feet are clapped together at top of movement

Reason for modification

Exercise would be contraindicated for persons with low bone density in the spine.

For sedentary workers, spine may already be in flexed position too much, albeit without muscle control.

Example modifications for individuals with insufficient core strength

- 4.5 Modified seated roll back
- 4.11 Supine lower back release
- 4.10 Shell/child pose stretch
- 4.7 Supine curl-up

Purpose

- Spine mobility

Reason for modification

Spine mobility can be achieved without momentum/speed and exercise would be contraindicated for persons with low bone density in the spine. Cervical vertebrae are in vulnerable position when weight bearing.

Example modifications for individuals with insufficient core strength

- 4.10 Shell/child pose stretch
- 5.15 Seated hamstring stretch

Control balance

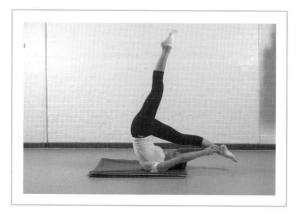

Perform scissor leg action in supine lying position. Knees can be bent to decrease leverage (5.3); then progress to extended lever.

Purpose

- Spine mobility
- Hamstring and hip flexor flexibility in open leg position
- Balance
- Pelvic and scapular stability
- Abdominal strength and endurance (progression from jack knife)

Reason for modification

Spine mobility can be achieved without weight-bearing movement. Exercise would be contraindicated for persons with low bone density in the spine. Cervical vertebrae and shoulder girdle are not designed for weight bearing. Stretches can be isolated.

Example modifications for individuals with insufficient core strength

- 5.12 Lying hamstring stretch
- 4.5 Modified seated roll back
- 4.11 Supine lower back release
- 4.3 Supine lying shoulder bridge
- 5.15 Seated hamstring stretch
- 6.3 Lying overhead arm float
- 5.4 Supine toe dips
- 5.3 Supine knee raise (alternating legs)

Push-up

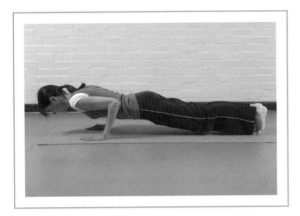

Purpose

- Upper body strength
- Abdominal strength
- Hamstring flexibility (when starting from standing position and bending forwards)

Reason for modification

Build strength and then exercise can be progressed to full position.

Example modifications for individuals with insufficient core strength

- 5.8 Prone lying leg raise
- 5.9 Gluteal bracing
- 5.5 Hands and knees leg raise
- 6.8 Hands and knee cat peddles
- 6.9 Hands and knees arm reach
- 6.13 Hands and knees to plank
- 6.14 Hands and knees press-up
- 5.15 Seated hamstring stretch (perform position standing when flexible)

Note: Those interested in developing their knowledge of these exercises should contact one of the schools listed at the end of this book. Each school will offer their own modifications and methods of progression.

GLOSSARY

Active stretching Contracting the opposite muscle to achieve a stretch. For example, relying on the strength of the hamstrings to lift the heel to the buttocks and achieve a quadriceps stretch.

Abduction Moving a body part away from the midline of the body, for example lifting the arm or leg out to the side, away from the body

Adduction Moving a body part back towards the midline of the body, for example lowering the arm or leg back towards the body from an abducted position

Anatomical position The position of the body when standing upright and erect, with feet positioned together and the palms of the hands facing forwards

Anterior Closer to the front of a structure or the body, for example the anterior superior iliac spine (ASIS) is at the front and top of the pelvis

Appendicular skeleton Its main role is to facilitate movement. It consists of the 126 bones of the arms, legs, hands, feet, pectoral/shoulder girdle, and pelvic girdle. The pelvic and shoulder girdle also have an integral role in supporting the body to maintain central/core stability.

Axial skeleton The main supportive structure of the body. It includes the skull or cranium, the vertebral column, the sternum and the ribcage (80 bones).

Ballistic stretching Bouncing at the end of the range of movement, which can result in muscle tears

Circumduction Moving a limb in a circular motion, for example the backstroke swimming action

Deep Further away from the surface of the body, for example multifidus is deeper than erector spinae

Depression Lowering the shoulder girdle downwards, for example sliding the shoulder blades down towards the lower back

Developmental stretching Performing a static stretch at the end of the range. Then taking the muscle beyond that range until the stretch reflex occurs again and holding at this increased ROM for an increased duration.

Directional terminology Terms used to explained the position of one body structure in relation to another, for example anterior, superior etc

Dynamic stretching Functional movements that take the muscle through the full range in a controlled manner, without excessive speed and momentum

Elevation Lifting the shoulder girdle upwards, for example raising the shoulders to the ears

Extension A straightening movement at the joint (for example, the knee or elbow), increasing the angle to return to the anatomical position

Flexibility The ability of the joints and muscles to move through their full potential range of movement

Flexion A bending movement at the joint (for example, the knee or elbow), decreasing the angle to bring the bones towards each other

Forced vital capacity The maximum volume of air moved through forceful inspiration and expiration

Frontal plane The plane that divides the body into front and back and affords movements such as abduction and adduction

Horizontal flexion Bringing the arms across the front of the body (horizontally), for example in hugging or wrapping arms around someone

Horizontal extension Taking the arms backwards from a horizontally flexed position, for example releasing a hug or drawing the elbows backwards from a chest press

Hyperextension Bending a joint backwards beyond the anatomical position of extension. Examples are locking out of the elbow or knee joints and excessive hollowing of the lumbar spine, as in lordosis.

Inferior Closer to the bottom or lower part of a structure, for example the lumbar vertebrae are inferior to the thoracic vertebrae

Isometric Static muscle contraction

Isotonic Moving muscle contraction consisting of shortening (lifting phase) and eccentric (lowering phase) muscle work

Lateral Closer to the outer side of a structure or the body and away from the midline, for example lateral rotation occurs by turning the hands away from the thighs

Lateral flexion and extension Bending the spine to one side and returning to straight, for example bending and straightening the spine or neck sideways

Maintenance stretching Stretching to maintain existing levels of flexibility

Medial Towards the midline or inner side of a structure or the body, for example medial rotation occurs by twisting the arms towards the thighs

Mobility The range of movement that exists around a joint

Passive stretching Assisting the opposite muscle to relax to achieve a stretch of the main muscle, for example holding the foot to perform a quadriceps stretch

Posterior Closer to the back of a structure or the body, for example the posterior superior iliac spine (PSIS) is at the back and top of the pelvis

Preparatory stretching Stretching to prepare muscles for activity (controversial area)

Proprioceptive neuromuscular facilitation (PNF) A method of stretching using a partner that exploits the relaxation response of the golgi tendon organ

Protraction and retraction Gliding movements forwards and backwards that occur at the shoulder girdle, for example rounding the shoulder girdle (protraction) and drawing back the shoulder girdle (retraction)

Residual volume The volume of air left in the lungs during maximal expiration

Rotation Turning or twisting a bone around its own long axis, for example trunk twists, neck twists, twisting the shoulder and hip inwards and outwards

Sagittal plane The plane that divides the body into right and left sides and affords movements such as flexion and extension

Static stretching Taking the muscle to the point of mild tension (stretch reflex) and holding still, allowing the muscle to relax

Stretching Exercises specifically targeted to relax and lengthen the muscles by moving the origin and insertion further apart

Stretch reflex A safety mechanism within the muscle that is activated when a muscle lengthens (usually at speed). The stretch reflex will contract the muscle (felt as a tension or, in extreme instances, as shaking) to prevent overstretching and damage to the muscle and surrounding tissues. The aim is to move slowly into stretch positions to reduce the effects of the stretch reflex.

Superficial Closer to the surface of the body, for example erector spinae is superficial to multifidus

Superior Closer to the top or upper part of a structure, for example the skull is superior to the shoulder girdle

Tidal volume The volume of air breathed in or out in any one breath

Transverse plane The plane that divides the body into top and bottom sections and affords movements such as rotation

REFERENCES AND RECOMMENDED READING

ACSM (2005) Guidelines for Exercise testing and Prescription. USA. Lippincott, Williams and Williams

Central YMCA Qualifications (2006), *Exercise and Fitness Knowledge Level 3*, CYQ.

Dale, B. & Roeber, J. (1984), *Exercises for Childbirth*, Century Hutchinson.

David Coultier, H. (2001), *Anatomy of Hatha Yoga: A Manual for Students, Teachers and Practitioners*, Body and Breath.

Department of Health (2004), *At Least Five a Week. Evidence on the Impact of Physical Activity and its Relationship to Health*, HMSO.

Department of Health (2004b), *Choosing Health: Making Healthier Choices Easier*, HMSO.

Department of Health (2005), *Choosing Activity: A Physical Activity Action Plan*, HMSO.

Devereux, G. (1998), *Dynamic Yoga*, Thorsons.

Drake, R. et al (2008), Gray's Atlas of Anatomy, Churchill Livingstone.

Fostater, M. & Manuel, J. (2002), *The Spiritual Teachings of Yoga*, Hodder and Stoughton.

Hately Aldous, S. (2005), *Anatomy and Asana: Preventing Yoga Injuries*, Functional Synergy Press.

Hately Aldous, S. (2005), *Anatomy and Asana: The Shoulder Girdle*, Functional Synergy Press.

Hately Aldous, S. (2005), *Anatomy and Asana: The Sacroiliac Joints*, Functional Synergy Press.

Hately Aldous, S. (2005), *Anatomy and Asana: The Knees*, Functional Synergy Press.

Hine, J. (1992), *Yang Tai Chi Chaun*, A & C Black.

Keane, S. (2005), *Pilates for Core Strength*, Greenwich Editions.

Latey, P. (2001), *Modern Pilates*, Allen & Unwin.

Lawrence, D. (2005), *The Complete Guide to Exercise to Music*, 2nd edition, A & C Black.

Lawrence, D. (2005), *The Complete Guide to Exercising Away Stress*, A & C Black.

Lawrence, D. & Barnett, L. (2006), *GP Referral Schemes*, A & C Black.

Merrithew, M. (2001), *STOTT Pilates: The Contemporary Approach*, Merrithew Corporation.

Norris, C. (1994), *Flexibility: Principles and Practice*, A & C Black.

Norris, C. (2001), *Abdominal Training*, A & C Black.

Northern Fitness and Education (2004a), *Modern Pilates Stage 1. Matwork Instructor Training Programme*, Northern Fitness and Education.

Northern Fitness and Education (2004b), *Modern Pilates Stage 2. Practitioner and Personal Trainer. Modern Approaches to Core Stability & Postural Alignment*, Northern Fitness and Education.

O'Byrne, S. (2006), *Yoga for the Core: Finding Stability in an Unstable Environment*, Functional Synergy.

Oliver, L. (1987), *Meditation and the Creative Imperative*, Dryad Press.

Palastanga, N., Field, D. & Soames, R. (1989), *Anatomy and Human Movement: Structure and Function*, Bath Press.

Pilates Method Alliance (2006), *Position Statement: On Pilates*.

REPs (2005), *REPs Journal*, Issue 3, Register of Exercise Professionals.

Robinson, L. et al (2000), *The Official Body Control Pilates Manual*, Macmillan.

Stone, R. & Stone, J. (1990), *Atlas of Skeletal Muscles*, McGraw-Hill.

Thompson, C. (1989), *Manual of Structural Kinesiology*, Times Mirror Mosby College Publications.

Tortura, G. & Anagnostakos, N. (1987), *Principles of Anatomy and Physiology,* 5th edition, Harper and Row.

Van Deurzan, A in Feltham, C & Horton, I (2000) Eds. *Handbook of Counselling and Psychotherapy.* UK. Sage Publications.

USEFUL WEBSITES

Body Control – Lynne Robinson
www.bodycontrol.co.uk/lynne.html

Alan Herdman
www.alanherdmanPilates.co.uk

Symmetry Fitness
www.symmetryfitness.com/history.html

Michael King
www.Pilates-institute.com

Moira Merrithew
www.stottPilates.com.media/releases/biomoira.html

Cherry Baker
www.modernPilates.co.uk
www.thestudioglossop.co.uk

Active Pilates – Jane Parsons
www.activePilates.co.uk

Dreas Reyneke
www.dreas.co.uk

Pilates Training Solutions
www.Pilatestrainingsolutions.co.uk

Pilates Foundation
www.Pilatesfoundation.com

Pilates Umbrella
www.Pilatesumbrella.co.uk

Pilates Method Alliance
www.Pilatesmethodalliance.org

Central YMCA Qualifications
www.cyq.org.uk

Chi Ball
www.chiball.com

Register of Exercise Professionals
www.exerciseregister.org

SkillsActive
www.skillsactive.com

Oriental Body Balance College
www.orientalbodybalance.co.uk

INDEX